Date Due	Date Due	Date Due	Date Due

This book should be returned on or before the last date shown above. It should be returned immediately if requested by the library. Fines are charged for overdue books.

An Essential Guide for Student Midwives: Preparing for Professional Practice

Edited by
Sue Jacob and Tina Lavender

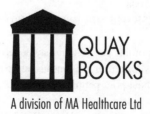

QUAY
BOOKS

A division of MA Healthcare Ltd

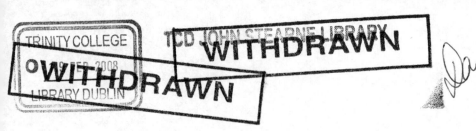

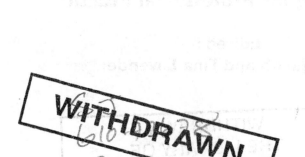

Quay Books Division, MA Healthcare Ltd, St Jude's Church, Dulwich Road, London
SE24 0PB

British Library Cataloguing-in-Publication Data
A catalogue record is available for this book

Printed by Ashford Colour Press, Gosport, Hants, PO13 0FW

Contents

Foreword   *Monica Thompson*   xi

Chapter 1   The statutes Governing the Role of the Midwife   13
                  Paul Lewis, Janine Davis

Chapter 2   Gaining Confidence and Competence as a Midwife   37
                  Rosaline Steele

Chapter 3   A Career in Midwifery   55
                  Pat R Donovan

Chapter 4   A Student Midwife's Experiences   71
                  in the 21st Century
                  Lisa McTavish

Chapter 5   The Paradox of Normal Childbirth: 83
                  a 21st Century Dialogue
                  Jane Walker

Chapter 6   Understanding Evidence-based   95
                  Midwifery Practice
                  Tina Lavender

Chapter 7   Does Litigation Influence Midwifery Practice?   117
                  Andrew Symon

Chapter 8   Changing Social and Political Constructs: 137
                  Impact on the Role of the Midwife
                  Carol Bates

Chapter 9   Feminist Perspectives in Midwifery   151
                  Carol Bates

Chapter 10   Conflict, Culture and Opportunities   161
                  for Midwives
                  Sue Jacob

Chapter 11   My Journey   181
                  Dame Lorna Muirhead

Index   *199*

Note

While the authors and publishers have made every effort, as far as is possible, to confirm the information in this book complies with the latest standards of practice and legislation, the authors and the publishers cannot take responsibility from any instances arising as a result of errors. Healthcare practice and knowledge are constantly changing and developing. Practitioners are encouraged to seek help where they are not competent to carry out a procedure.

Contributors

Carol Bates
Carol is Midwifery Education and Practice Consultant. Carol became a midwife in 1967. She was Director of Midwifery Education at University College Hospitals, London, from 1992 to 1996, following which she worked in the Education Department at the Royal College of Midwives until 2006. Carol Bates is an experienced clinical midwife and educationalist and has published widely on all aspects of midwifery practice. She also has a particular interest in risk management. During the course of her career Carol Bates has represented midwifery on many multidisciplinary committees.

Janine Davis
Janine has been a midwife in practice and education for over twenty-five years and holds a Master of Science degree in midwifery practice. She is currently Senior Lecturer and programme leader for post registration midwifery programmes at Bournemouth University. She continues to engage with practice through her link midwife teacher role and it is experienced in the needs of student midwives and their mentors in respect of the preregistration midwifery programme. Janine has a keen interest in the history of the midwife and the professional regulation.

Pat Donovan
Pat is Lead Midwife for Education at the University of Central Lancashire. Pat qualified as a Nurse and Midwife in London in the 1970s and initially practised midwifery in Israel and also London. On qualifying as a teacher she moved into midwifery education, where she has been for the last 20 years, working in the West Country and South coast. Her research areas are education, embryology, and research methodology and she has published in the area of research methodology, key skills and general midwifery.

Sue Jacob
Sue is Student Services Advisor at the Royal College of Midwives. Sue worked as a midwifery lecturer prior to joining the Royal College of Midwives in 1995, and has extensive experience in all aspects of midwifery education and practice at policy and planning services level. Key aspects of her teaching role include developing, delivering and evaluating pre-registration and postqualification and return to practice education programmes. Her international work includes organising visits for overseas visitors to the RCM. She was a co-facilitator of 'training the teachers' Indonesia Safe Motherhood project. Sue is a proactive member of the medical and non-medical RCM International Forum.

Professor Tina Lavender
Tina is Professor in Midwifery and Women's Health at the University of Central Lancashire and leads a stream of research on the experiences, expectations and outcomes of maternity care. Tina is an Honorary Consultant Midwife at the Liverpool Women's Foundation Trust, where she leads a programme of clinically based research centring on optimizing normal birth. Tina is also committed to working internationally, through partnerships with groups such as the East Central and South African College of Nursing. She is a member of the White Ribbon Alliance for Safe Motherhood and the National Clinical FGM group. Tina is a member of the Cochrane Collaboration, responsible for a number of Systematic Reviews and is Joint Editor-in-Chief of the British Journal of Midwifery and Associate Editor of the African Journal of Midwifery. She is also a current Honorary Fellow of the Royal College of Midwives.

Professor Paul Lewis
Paul is the Associate Dean of Midwifery, Rehabilitation and Health Sciences at Bournemouth University and leads its provision of midwifery education programmes and post graduate midwifery studies. Over the last 10 years he has been a Council member on both the UKCC and Nursing and Midwifery Council. He was elected to the current NMC and chairs both the Statutory Midwifery and Conduct and Competence Committees. Throughout his career he has remained clinically engaged. He is an instructor and faculty member of ALSO (UK); a Supervisor of Midwives at Poole NHS Trust and a Member of RCM Council.

Lisa McTavish
Lisa is a student midwife studying in Glasgow. Before commencing her midwifery programme Lisa worked for 10 years as a Registered Nurse for Learning Disabilities in Ayrshire.

Dame Lorna Muirhead
Dame Lorna Muirhead is Her Majesty's Lord-Lieutenant of Merseyside and the Immediate Past President of The Royal College of Midwives. Lorna's professional life has been in Clinical Midwifery, which spanned the years between 1965-2005. During that time, she lived through many changes within the NHS and huge philosophical changes regarding childbirth amongst midwives and the women for whom they care. Dame Lorna is often invited to air those views at study days and in debate as indeed she has been in the chapter of this book.

Rosaline Steele
Rosaline is Education Consultant and Fellow of the Higher Education

Academy. An experienced midwife educator with a particular interest in the continuing education of midwives, Rosaline has been influential in the development of midwifery education at a local and national level. She is particularly proud of her work at national level, in which she facilitated education programmes which broadened midwives understanding of antenatal testing for HIV. Rosaline successfully led one of the fist wave developments of the direct entry pre-registration midwifery programme in a period when those programmes were not the norm. Rosaline's current research interests are in the development of midwifery professionalism and the generation of new knowledge from practice.

Andrew Symon
Andrew is a Senior Lecturer at the School of Nursing and Midwifery, University of Dundee. Andrew qualified in 1986, following which he worked in both Scotland and Kenya as a midwife. After his first degree in Social Policy and Law he worked as a research midwife in Edinburgh, then parttime as a midwife in Perth. He completed his PhD in 1997. He has published two books based on this research, and has edited two more on clinical risk management. Research interests include the assessment of quality of life, independent midwifery, and nutrition during and after pregnancy.

Jane Walker
Jane is Consultant Midwife Homerton University Hospital, Hackney, North East London, and Supervisor of Midwives. She is working with Hackney Council, the local PCT and with local voluntary agencies leading a programme of work for reducing infant mortality. Jane has been a midwife since 1981. She was previously a lecturer in midwifery at City University, London, and has also been a senior midwifery manager. She has been project leader at the Edgware Birth Centre during the early years and through its important evaluation period. She has travelled extensively in UK and Europe lecturing about this subject. Her most recent research activity was a study of women's attitudes towards their behaviour in labour.

Foreword

A much welcomed, balancing, practical and insightful resource has finally arrived. This is a unique book and valuable guide for students as it not only provides essential information for them but also gives an honest, personalised and critical reflection of midwifery experiences across the UK.

This work is organised to cover the key themes of education, regulation, evidence and practice, as well as tracing political, social and cultural constructs that have hindered and helped the scope and sphere of practice. A refreshing inclusion is a number of chapters to raise the feminist and political consciousness amongst students during their formative years in the profession.

Increasingly, maternity services are responsive to divergent, political and policy agendas across the four UK countries and so are transforming to include a variety of providers and path-finder models. The resultant challenges and conflicts for midwives and the dilemmas these pose have been explored effectively by the contributors to this book.

Mindful of its key readership, the editors have included 'activity boxes' at the end of each chapter to stimulate reflection and creative thinking and so further challenge enquiring minds. The inclusion of useful website sources of evidence, model templates, and the application of key legislation to the role of the midwife are welcome additions to the student toolbox.

The influence of early key role models and inspirational mentors in shaping midwifery practice and the value of professional networks sustaining it are well articulated in its pages. For this alone, the book is essential reading for all student midwives.

Monica Thompson
Programme Director (Midwifery and Women's Health)
NHS Education for Scotland

CHAPTER 1

The Statutes Governing the Role of the Midwife

Paul Lewis, Janine Davis

An essential aspect of professional practice is to understand and have insight into the immediate legal requirements, rules and regulations which determine our work and the wider legislation that shapes and directs our practice as providers of health and social care. In particular, to recognise the duties, obligations and responsibilities that being a midwife demands. At all times, we are expected to act in the best interests of the public we serve, as well as upholding the good name and standing of our profession. Like all members of our wider society we are expected to respect and uphold the laws of the land but in addition, to demonstrate the qualities of kindness, caring and consideration that is embodied in the role of the midwife. These qualities are integral to the expectations that the public have of us as responsible, individual members of a regulated professional body. They are part and parcel of our essential requirements of care and of vital importance to those who call upon our midwifery skills and knowledge. Without demonstrating these values and abiding by our standards, rules and codes of conduct, we risk losing the confidence and support of the wider public; who ultimately validate the positions we hold as midwives within our local communities and the society in which we live.

Yet the legal framework that govern the role of the midwife is for many student midwives, as well as some qualified practitioners, an area of professional practice that take second place to the acquisition of skills, knowledge and personal experiences that more overtly define who and what we are as clinicians. Nevertheless, without knowledge of the principles and statutes that govern the role of the midwife, we are at constant risk of breaching the codes, rules and regulations that seek to ensure the required standards of practice and the imperative of public protection. This can sometimes end with catastrophic results, not only for your own personal and professional esteem but also to the detriment of those to whom you are morally, legally and professionally bound; the mothers, babies and families in your care.

This chapter sets the statutes governing the role of the midwife. The basis of this chapter is to help you to understand the legal and professional duties and statutes that student midwives seeking entry to the professional register will have to meet. This is in order to ensure safe and effective practice that best protects the public and maintains the good standing of the midwifery profession.

Most of you reading this chapter will no doubt be excited and perhaps overwhelmed by the opportunities and challenges with which you are now confronted as you begin your education to become midwives. The short years ahead will be demanding, but the privileges which come with being a student of midwifery and future registered midwife have not been without struggle and adversity. Our success today, in respect of professional self-regulation, is founded on the achievements, hard work and the heartfelt desire of those that preceded us to improve the lot of mothers and midwives. This chapter is a foundation which will hopefully help you to better understand your professional responsibilities; it is a beginning not an end to your learning.

A Brief History

The historical landmark in the history of the midwifery profession was the passing of the first Midwives Act in 1902. This had far-reaching implications for every midwife in England and Wales. Subsequent legislation led to the passing of Midwives Acts in Scotland (1915) and Northern Ireland (1922). All sought to secure better training for midwives and to regulate their practise for the protection of the public. The 1902 Act established the Central Midwives Board (CMB) as our first regulatory body and also initiated the beginnings of what was to later become Statutory Supervision of Midwives (Kirkham, 1995; Halksworth et al, 2000). Over time, the 1902 Midwives Act was amended and added to with subsequent acts in 1918, 1926, 1934, 1936 and 1950. In 1951 the final Midwives Act consolidated all previous acts (Ackerman, 2004).

With the passing of the Midwives' Act in 1902 and the creation of the CMB, midwifery in England and Wales became a self regulated profession for the first time. However, such regulation was embryonic and much has changed over the intervening years in both our approach to the practice of midwifery, the provision of maternity care and the mores and values of our society in the 21st Century.

The CMB remained in place for nearly 80 years until it gave way to a new regulator, the United Kingdom Central Council (UKCC), which was established with the passing of the Nurses, Midwives and Health Visitors Act 1979 (Davies and Beach, 2000). A mere 18 years later, we experienced further change in professional regulation with Parliament passing the Nursing and Midwifery Order (2001) (DH, 2002a), which quickly led to the demise of the UKCC and the four National Boards (Lewis, 2007). The Nursing and Midwifery Council (NMC) was established in 2002.

Changes in Society and the Law

As a student midwife it is all too easy to focus on the work at hand, that of 'becoming a midwife'. This can lead to a very narrow perception of what is expected of us and it is essential that you recognise the wider implications of social change and the imperatives which arise out of the concomitant changes in the law. As Sarah Roch, a former chair of the UKCC Statutory Midwifery Committee stated in her foreword to 'The Midwife and Society' (Symonds and Hunt, 1996):

> *'Understanding the sociological context in which [midwives] practise midwifery is also a prerequisite for attaining that proper political perspective, without which the art and science of midwifery will not prosper or develop to meet the ever-changing needs of the public we all serve'.*

Sarah Roch, 1996

Tracing an Act of Parliament can be tricky but the use of the internet makes this less problematic and it is a useful exercise to access, explore and begin to understand the complexities of the law and legal system within the UK. The House of Commons Information Office provide fact sheets which can be accessed over the internet which should assist you in tracing Acts of Parliament (see *Resources* section at the end of this chapter).

As a student of midwifery you may begin to wonder about the sense of this considering all the other demands that you already face in your pre-registration programme of education. However, this underpinning knowledge is essential to a better understanding of the rights and responsibilities required of us as individuals, employees, employers and professional practitioners working within the field of health and social care in the 21st century.

The Structure and Functions of the NMC

The Nursing and Midwifery Order 2001 brought an end to the UKCC and the four National Boards and established the NMC as the regulator of the two professions of Nursing and Midwifery. This secondary legislation is located in the 1999 Health Act, Part III, Section 60(1), which sets out the 'Regulation of health care and associated professions'. This states that Her Majesty may by Order in Council make provision:

(a) modifying the regulation of any profession to which subsection (2) applies, so far as appears to Her to be necessary or expedient for the purpose of securing or improving the regulation of the profession or the services which the profession provides or to which it contributes,

(b) regulating any other profession which appears to Her to be concerned (wholly or partly) with the physical or mental health of individuals and to require regulation in pursuance of this section.

The NMC and its appointed Council took up office in April 2002. The Order created the 'body corporate' known as the Nursing and Midwifery Council and defined its principal function, which was to:

'...establish from time to time standards of education, training, conduct and performance for nurses and midwives and to ensure the maintenance of those standards'

NMC, 2001: Part II, 3 (2)

The main objective of the Council in exercising its functions is to:

'...safeguard the health and well-being of persons using or needing the services of registrants'

NMC, 2001: Part II, 3 (4)

The primary duty of the NMC is to protect the public, and this is achieved by:

- Establishing and maintaining a register of all nurses, midwives and specialist community public health nurses
- Setting standards for education and training, leading to entry to the register
- Setting standards for conduct, performance and professional updating for maintenance on the register
- Applying conditions or sanctions against registrants or removing them from the register in order to protect the public.

The Nursing and Midwifery Order 2001 makes interesting reading and clearly sets out the line of accountability that the NMC has to the Privy Council. They are required to consult the Queen's Privy Council or such persons as the Privy Council designate at least once in each calendar year on the way in which it proposes to exercise its functions (NMC 2001, Part II, 3 (7)).

The Council itself is made up of 35 members; a designate registered nurse, midwife and specialist community public health nurse are elected from each of the four countries of the UK. An alternate registrant member is also elected in each of these categories, and although they are unable to vote when their designate member is present, they are involved in all other aspects of the Council including membership and chairmanship of the Statutory Committees.

There are 11 lay members of the NMC, and each is appointed on merit and with a view to the skills and experience they can bring to professional regulation. The voting members of the NMC comprise the 11 lay members and 12 designate registrant members or their alternate if they are not able to be present. This gives a total of 23 votes that can be cast in Council on any matter which needs to be decided, with a professional majority of just one vote. This increased lay membership is in direct contrast to that of NMC's predecessors (the Central Midwives Board (CMB) the General Nursing Council (GNC) and the UKCC), all of whom has either minimal or no lay member on their Councils.

This was an important and significant change in professional regulation and cuts across all healthcare regulators. There is now both the political and professional will to more fully engage with public participation and involve lay membership in the regulation of the health professions. It comes in response to a lack of public confidence in the professions to regulate themselves, in the wake of several high profile cases such as the Bristol Heart Inquiry (DH, 2002), the Shipman Inquiry and those of the Ayling, Neale and Kerr/Haslam Inquiries (HMG, 2007a). All make salutary reading, but as the Secretary of State suggests:

'It is all too easy to focus on the incompetent or malicious practice of individuals, and seek to build a system from that starting point instead of recognising that excellent health professionals far outnumber the few who let patients down substantially - we must recall the hundreds of thousands of extraordinary individuals who dedicate themselves impeccably to their patients every day'.

HMG 2007b:1

'Most health professionals meet high standards routinely and have a lifelong appetite to be even better. That professionalism is an unquantifiable asset to our society, which rules, regulations and systems must support, not inhibit.'

HMG 2007b:1

The primary duty of the NMC is not to punish registrants for wrong doing, but to establish standards that will facilitate excellence, protect the public and promote the good standing of nursing and midwifery. The NMC achieves this through its Council and several important Strategic and

Statutory Committees, which have been established to progress the work, development and direction of the NMC.

In considering the statutes that govern the role of the midwife, the Council and its four Statutory Committees set most if not all of the codes, rules and regulations that direct our professional practice. It is not the intention of this Chapter to go into these in detail, as such Codes are available free of charge from the NMC; they make compelling reading and all students of midwifery should acquire the following in the first few days or weeks of their professional education. Make sure that you have a copy of:

- *Standards of Proficiency for Pre-registration Midwifery Education* (NMC, 2004a)
- *Midwives Rules and Standards* (NMC, 2004b)
- *Code of Professional Conduct: Standards for conduct, performance and ethics* (NMC, 2004c)
- *Standards for the Preparation and Practice of Supervisors of Midwives* (NMC, 2006).

It is also possible to get more detailed advice through the NMC's Professional Advisory Service (see *Resources* section at the end of this chapter). Importantly, your Higher Education Institution (HEI) will also provide recommended reading lists within their validated midwifery programme, which will direct you to the pertinent literature that supports the learning outcomes in your modules/units of education. The responsibility for making the most of these opportunities rests with yourselves as students, and is a forerunner to the personal and professional responsibilities and autonomy upon which your future practice as a registered midwife is predicated.

The Statutory Committees

The four Statutory Committees of the NMC are:

- The Investigation Committee
- The Health Committee
- The Conduct and Competence Committee
- The Midwifery Committee.

The first three are known as practice committees and deal with all issues pertaining to fitness to practise, ethics and other matters (NMC 2001, Part V, 21 (1)). The Nursing and Midwifery Order 2001 states that the Council shall:

(a) establish and keep under review the standards of conduct, performance and ethics expected of registrants and prospective registrants and give them such guidance on these matters as it sees fit: and

(b) establish and keep under review effective arrangements to protect the public from persons whose fitness to practise is impaired.

Allegations may be brought against registrants when their fitness to practise is impaired by reason of:

(i) misconduct

(ii) lack of competence

(iii) a conviction or caution in the United Kingdom for a criminal offence, or a conviction elsewhere for an offence which, if committed in England and Wales would constitute a criminal offence

(iv) his/her physical or mental health, or

(v) a determination by a body in the United Kingdom responsible under any enactment for the regulation of a health or social care profession to the effect that his fitness to practise is impaired, or a determination by a licensing body elsewhere to the same effect (NMC 2001, Part V, 22 (1a))

(vi) an entry in the register relating to him/her had been fraudulently procured or incorrectly made (NMC 2001, Part V, 21 (1b)).

The membership of the strategic fitness to practise committees of the NMC is made up of the Council members, alongside an appointed Registered Medical Practitioner. However, the panels that deal directly with the proceedings brought by the Council against registrants, have in the past been made up of Council members as well as lay and professional panellists; and where the health of the respondent if in question, a register medical practitioner.

Since 31st September 2007, and in keeping with the Government's White Paper '*Trust, Assurance and Safety – The Regulation of Health Professionals in the 21st Century*' (DH, 2007b), a separation of function has been brought about and Council members of the NMC are no longer able to sit on any fitness to practise panel, although they remain engaged indirectly through their involvement in the strategic committees. Where the health of the respondent is in question the committee will include a registered medical practitioner.

The Midwifery Committee

The Midwifery Committee is of vital importance to our profession and provides the necessary leadership and direction in a Council in which midwives are outnumbered 2:1 by members of the nursing profession. The right to have a midwifery committee within the structure of the NMC was not automatic and as in times past, this privilege had to be fought for and has been hard won.

The role of the Midwifery Committee is to advise the Council, at the Council's request or otherwise, on any matters affecting midwifery (NMC 2001, Part VIII, 41(1)). Equally, the Council is required to:

> *'...consult the Midwifery Committee on the exercise of its functions in so far as it affects midwifery including any proposals to make rules under article 42'.*

NMC 2001, Part VIII, 41 (2)

The Midwifery Committee is made up of the eight midwives elected to Council from the four countries of the UK. In addition, there are lay members of the Council who, either through involvement in childbirth organisations such as AIMS or the NCT, are appointed to be members of the Committee. In addition to this, lay and registrant non-Council members may be appointed or co-opted to assist the Committee in its deliberations and decisions. Currently, the eight midwife members of Council, two lay Council members and three non-Council lay members make up the membership of the midwifery committee.

The Code of Professional Conduct

The introduction to the Code sets out its purpose, which is to inform the professions of the standard of conduct required of them in the exercise of their professional accountability and practice; and to inform the public, other professions and employers of the standard that they can expect of a Registered Practitioner (NMC, 2004c).

The Code is the principal guidance of the NMC which all registered nurses and midwives are required to follow, regardless of where they work or for whom they work. It is against these standards that the acts and omissions of registrants and prospective registrants will be judged. As such, they are of vital importance and provide the touchstone against which midwives can practice safely and effectively.

The Code has been through a number of iterations over the years in order for it to remain relevant to current practice and be readily understood by registrants. The current Code of professional conduct was published by the NMC in April 2002 and came into effect on 1 June 2002. In August 2004 an addendum was published and the Code of professional conduct had its name changed to *The NMC Code of Professional Conduct: Standards for Conduct, Performance and Ethics*. All references to 'nurses, midwives and health visitors' were replaced by 'nurses, midwives and specialist community public health nurses'. A new section on Indemnity Insurance was also included. The updated version of the code was published in November 2004 (NMC, 2004c). Recently, the NMC consulted on a new version of the Code to ensure it remains relevant, provides greater understanding and is easier to use. A wide range of stakeholders and members of the professions were engaged in the consultation.

It is vitally important that you not only know, but understand the content and intent of this important document: The code is currently divided into nine sections (see *Table 1*).

All aspects of the Code apply equally to midwives, nurses and specialist community public health nurses and is therefore, essential reading. However, the recent addition of Section 9 has particular resonance for midwives with direct consequences for the work of self-employed midwives in independent

Table 1. Sections of the current Code and proposed sections of the new Code

The NMC Code of Professional Conduct: Standards for Conduct, Performance and Ethics	NMC Code under consultation
1. Introduction and intent of the Code	Section A: 'Make the care of people your first concern,
2. Respect the patient or client as an individual	treating them as individuals and respecting their dignity'
3. Obtain consent before you give any treatment or care	Section B: 'Work with others to protect and promote the health and well being of those in your
4. Co-operate with others in the team	care, their families and carers, and the wider community'
5. Protect confidential information	
	Section C: 'Provide a high
6. Maintain your professional knowledge and competence	standard of practice and care at all times'
7. Be trustworthy	Section D: 'Be open and honest, act with integrity and uphold
8. Act to identify and minimise the risk to patients and clients	the reputation of your profession'
9. Indemnity insurance	

practice. Section 9 recommends that a registered midwife has professional indemnity insurance in the event of claims of professional negligence. The NHS employers accept vicarious liability for the negligent acts and/ or omissions of their employees, however it is not extended to activities undertaken outside the registrant's employment. Independent midwives are self-employed and as such, are personally responsible for obtaining their own indemnity insurance. Midwives employed by an agency need to clarify their position with that employer. Midwives who have not secured professional indemnity insurance must inform their clients, as this has implications should a claim of professional negligence be made.

What Does the Code Mean to You as a Midwife?

As a registered midwife you are personally accountable for your practice. Student midwives need to work towards this ideal under the direction of their named mentor. Incrementally and increasingly throughout their pre-registration programme, student midwives will be required to take on additional responsibilities and decision-making. This is delegated to you by a registered midwife and will enable you to work towards achieving you professional requirements through direct and indirect supervision.

In caring for patients and clients, you must respect the patient or client as an individual, obtain consent before you give any treatment or care, protect confidential information and cooperate with others in the team (NMC, 2004c). Women and their families are central to the role and responsibilities of the midwife and it is in their interests, that we are duty bound. It is not acceptable to impose care which is against their wishes in order that the organisation may benefit or work more efficiently. Choice is a fundamental aspect of maternity care and the midwife and student midwife should do all in their power to support women in their choices, ensuring these are made from an informed position and that the women and her family are aware of the benefits and the risks associated with any course of action or omission.

Information given to the mother and/or recorded in her maternity record, should be for the sole purpose of providing her with care. Recently the NMC issued guidance on the ownership of midwifery records (NMC Circular 02/2007). These should be fully understood by all members of the midwifery profession. The importance and purpose of good record keeping should never be underestimated and as such, the following four paragraphs are taken directly from the above NMC circular and are cross referenced to the relevant Midwives Rules (NMC, 2004b).

Midwives are required to keep, as contemporaneously as is reasonable, continuous and detailed records of observations made, care and medicines given and any form of pain relief administered by her by the midwife to the woman or baby (NMC, 2004b). Contemporaneous records are made for the benefit of both the woman and the midwife; the woman so that she can be an active participant in deciding and directing the care she wishes to receive, and the midwife to ensure clear, written communication with other members of the healthcare team regarding her decision-making (and to help the midwife should any allegations be made against her). It is often the case that women carry their own maternity records (or have a shadow set) and it is usual that all necessary information is contained within these records.

When a midwife transfers a woman into a maternity unit from home or from one maternity unit to another, her records, with a detailed account of recent events, need to accompany the woman so that staff in the receiving unit can provide timely and appropriate care. This is in line with the principle of sharing records with other members of the healthcare team (NMC, 2004a). This principle equally applies to self-employed midwives and those employed by an organisation, and not to do so could place the midwife in breach of her professional duty and for self-employed midwives, possible contractual duty to the woman (NMC Circular 2007a).

The Code requires you to maintain your professional knowledge and competence, be trustworthy and to act at all times to identify and minimise risk to patients and clients. These are the shared values of all the health care regulatory bodies in the UK (NMC, 2004c), and as such there should be no difficulties in achieving consensus with other professions involved in maternity services and the provision of care to women and their families.

Standards of Proficiency for Pre-registration Midwifery Education

The NMC is required to establish and maintain a register of qualified nurses and midwives, and from time to time establish standards of proficiency to be met by applicants to different parts of the register, being the standards it considers necessary for safe and effective practice.

The proficiencies required of the student midwife are codified within both European as well as UK legislation and have been guided by the definition of a midwife, which was adopted by the International Confederation of Midwives (ICM) in 2005. This supersedes the ICM 'Definition of a Midwife' 1972 and its amendments of 1990. The definition reads as follows:

'A midwife is a person who, having been regularly admitted to a midwifery educational programme, duly recognised in the country in which it is located, has successfully completed the prescribed course of studies in midwifery and has acquired the requisite qualifications to be registered and/or licensed to practise midwifery.

'The midwife is recognised as a responsible and accountable professional who works in partnership with women to give the necessary support, care and advice during pregnancy, labour and the postpartum period, to conduct births on the midwife's own responsibility and to provide care for the newborn and the infant. This care includes preventative measures, the promotion of normal birth, the detections of complications in mother and child, the accessing of medical care or other appropriate assistance and the carrying out of emergency measures.'

ICM, 2005

The NMC's standards of proficiency for pre-registration midwifery education are set out in five sections as listed below:

- Section 1: Standards for pre-registration programmes
- Section 2: Standards for the Lead Midwife for Education
- Section 3: Standards for admission to and continued participation in programmes
- Section 4: Standards for the structure and nature of programmes
- Section 5: Standards for education to achieve the NMC standards of proficiency

Along with the 15 standards contained within these sections there are also guiding principles. These establish the philosophy and values underpinning the NMC's requirements for programmes leading to entry to the midwives' part of the register and should be reflected in the midwifery programmes (NMC, 2004a).

These are significant in determining the approach to care that all midwives should adhere to. In supporting students both teachers and mentors in practice should recognise that their education will:

- Demonstrate a women-centred approach to care based on partnership, which respects the individuality of the woman and her family. The use of the word 'family' refers to significant others, as identified by the woman.
- Promote ethical and non-discriminatory practices
- Reflect the quality dimension of care through the setting and maintenance of appropriate standards
- Develop the concept of lifelong learning in students, encompassing key skills including communications and teamwork
- Take account of the changing culture and context of midwifery practice
- Be based upon the best available evidence.

The pre-registration proficiencies are kept under review, and recent changes that the NMC Statutory Midwifery Committee is seeking to introduce are those of 'midwifery essential skills clusters' (ESC), which will be linked to points of progression between different academic levels. These, put simply, will require student midwives to demonstrate to the satisfaction of their 'sign off mentor' that they have met the required standard for their level of education and training. The ESC will require the student to be proficient in the areas of:

- The initial consultation between the woman and the midwife
- Communication
- Normal labour and birth
- Initiation and continuance of breastfeeding
- Medicines management.

The programme providers will need to determine how these are used, incorporated and assessed, and they will be linked to progression points within the midwifery programme. Academic standards have to be achieved and confirmed within 12 weeks of entering the next academic level.

Midwives Rules and Standards

The NMC Order 2001 requires the NMC to set rules and standards for midwifery. These include standards for the Local Supervising Authorities who are responsible for the function of statutory supervision of midwives (NMC 2004b). The NMC midwives rules form the requirements for registration and practice and are grounded in legislation. It is important that you study, learn and remember the rules so that the effectively inform your practise and work as a midwife.

There are 16 rules, which include interpretation, guidance and instruction on practice and supervision of midwifery. Rules 1 and 2 cover the commencement date and the interpretation of terms and expressions that apply to midwifery and its governance. Rules 3, 4, 5, 10, 11, 12, 13, 14, and 15 apply to the appointment and role of a supervisor and the functions of the local supervising authority. Rules 6, 7, 8 and 9 are related directly to midwifery practice. Rules 3, 6, 7 and 9 have been expanded later in the chapter to assist the student midwife to appreciate their relevance in ensuring safe practice and protecting the public.

The NMC (2004d) requires a student, as well as a qualified midwife, to declare all and any convictions or police cautions as well as illness or disability, which might adversely affect their ability to practise safely and effectively. The student midwife is required to submit a self-declaration on successful completion of the pre-registration programme, prior to entry to the NMC register (NMC 2004 [Rule 5 (1) (a)]). The declaration has to be supported by the Lead Midwife for Education [Rule 6 (1) (a) (ii)]. Students who fail to maintain the standards of conduct and behaviour expected of a future midwife may well be denied such support and be denied access to the midwifery profession where an individual's good standing is important to maintain public trust and confidence.

Examples of actions which would jeopardise your chances of a good character reference include acting fraudulently; altering educational or clinical records which brings into question their honesty and integrity; attempting to pervert the course of common justice by misleading the police or relevant authorities; deliberately misleading or misrepresenting themselves for personal gain; or receiving a police caution or conviction for a criminal offence.

> *'Applicants must demonstrate that they have good health and good character, sufficient for safe and effective practice as a midwife, on entry to, and for continued participation in, programmes leading to registration with the NMC'*

> NMC, 2004d

Rule 3 – Notification of Intention to Practise

This is an annual requirement for all qualified midwives on the NMC register who meet the practice requirements and intend to practise as a midwife in a given area:

1   If a midwife intends either to be in attendance upon a woman or baby during the antenatal, intranatal or postnatal period or to hold a post for which a midwifery qualification is required she shall give notice in accordance with paragraph (2).
2   A midwife shall give notice under paragraph (1) to each local supervising authority in whose area she intends to practise or continue to practise –
    a)   before commencing to practise there; and thereafter
    b)   in respect of each period of 12 months beginning on a date which the Council shall specify from time to time.
3   Notwithstanding the provisions of paragraph (2), the notice to be given under paragraph (1) may, in an emergency, be given after the time when she commences to practise provided that it is given within 48 hours of that time.

A notice to be given under this rule shall contain such particulars and be in such form as the Council may from time to time specify.

Rule 6 - Responsibility and Sphere of Practice

This rule lays parameters and boundaries of the role for midwives as practitioners of the normal childbirth. This can be translated into not providing any care, or undertaking any treatment, for which the midwife has not received education and training except in an emergency. The midwife is expected to call such qualified health professional as may have the necessary skills and experience to assist her in the provision of care that is outside her sphere of practice.

Rule 7 – Administration of Medicines

A practising midwife is expected to supply and administer those medicines, including analgesics when she has received the appropriate training as to their use, dosage and methods of administration. If a practising midwife has completed a recognised prescribing course, she is also entitled to prescribe within the limits of her competency to do so.

The impending requirement for medicine management skills at the end of the first year and third year of a pre-registration midwifery programme as part of the Essential Skills Cluster (ESC) will mean that these aspects of practice will take on greater priority.

Rule 9 – Records

Records and record keeping is an area of professional practice which is fraught with difficulties. The needs of the woman are central to your care but in order to ensure her wellbeing and an accurate record of the care she has received, a midwife needs to keep as contemporaneously as is reasonable, continuous and detailed records if observations made, care given and medicines and any form of pain relief administered by her to a woman or baby (Rule 9.1). You should make continuous and detailed notes on the following:

- What is happening — observations and assessment
- What action is required — plan of care
- What you action you have taken — further observations, care and treatment
- To what effect — evaluation of the care on the wellbeing of the mother and baby

Good record-keeping is a skill that requires practice and should never be just be about ticking boxes; it is a legal requirement and we should all strive to provide in written or electronic form. Entries should be documented in a manner which is accurate, concise, legible and clearly signed.

When a midwife transfers a woman into a maternity unit from home or from one maternity unit to another, her records, with a detailed account of recent events, need to accompany the woman so that staff in the receiving unit can provide timely and appropriate care.

This equally applies to self-employed midwives and those employed by an organisation and not to do so could place the midwife in breach of her professional duty and for self-employed midwives, possible contractual duty to the woman.

From time to time the Midwifery Committee issues guidelines to midwives on critical aspects of practice and education which are published as NMC circulars. It is important to read published NMC Circulars and checking their website for further Circulars. The following NMC Circulars address important aspects of midwifery practice:

- NMC Circular (2006a) Midwives and Home Birth
- NMC Circular (2006b) Midwives and Exposure Prone Procedures
- NMC Circular (2006a) Ownership and Sharing of Midwifery Records
- NMC Circular (2007b) The care of babies born alive at the threshold of viability
- NMC Circular (2007c) Review of pre-registration midwifery education

Statutory Supervision of Midwives

As students progress through their pre-registration programme the issues around risk management and clinical governance arrangements to support practice will become more apparent. Statutory supervision of midwives is one of the key components of risk management in maternity services.

The Midwives Rules and Standards include guidelines to the appointment, duties, and responsibilities of supervisors of midwives (SoM), Local Supervising Midwifery Officers (LSAMOs) and Local Supervising Authorities (LSAs).

Every practising midwife is allocated a SoM; increasingly universities are allocating a SoM to be responsible for a cohort of student midwives. This approach simulates the named supervisor model which all midwives in the UK are privileged to have.

It also establishes a relationship between the supervisor and the students, some of whom on qualification seek employment within the Trust and require a named supervisor.

Activity 1

1. Outline the aims and achievements of the 1902 Midwives Act, the 1979 Nurse, Midwives and Health Visitors Act, and the Nursing and Midwifery Order 2001.

2. In keeping with your studies, try to attend if possible, a fitness to practise hearing of the Conduct and Competence Committee, which are open to the public. See if you can determine the makeup of the panel, the key individuals involved and the roles which may be played out in a fitness to practise hearing.

3. List the sanctions that a fitness to practise panel of the NMC is entitled to make and discuss the possible impact and implications of these.

4. Review the NMC circulars that are current on the NMC website and identify those which have direct relevance to the day-to-day provision of midwifery education and practice.

5. Within Standard 15 of the *Standards of Proficiency for Pre-registration Midwifery Education* (NMC, 2004a), identify the standards of education you need to achieve in order to be proficient within each of the following domains:
    - Effective midwifery practice (n=15)
    - Professional and ethical practice (n= 8)
    - Developing the individual midwife and others (n=2)
    - Achieving quality care through evaluation and research (n=4)

6. Identify an event in the care of a mother, which is outside of the parameters of normality and occurs either in the antenatal, intrapartum or postpartum periods. What action would you take and how would this relate to Rule 6 of the *Midwives Rules and Standards* (NMC, 2004c)?

7. As a student midwife you are asked to administer 100 milligrams of pethidine to a woman in labour. List the process you would take and the legal and practice requirements for safe and effective administration.

8. Under the direction of your mentor, review the records of a woman and identify the strengths and weaknesses of the record. In what way might they be misinterpreted or misdirect the care of others?

Additional Guidance and Legislation

There is a plethora of additional legislation that influences and governs midwives' practice and is becoming increasingly relevant to deliver a service that is safe, transparent, accountable and protects the public from any harm. Relevant legislation that you should read at some point during your studies (and keep refreshed during your practice), includes:

- Births and Deaths Registration Act 1953
- Congenital Disabilities (Civil Liability) Act 1976
- The Rehabilitation of Offenders Act 1976
- The Medicines (Pharmacy and General Sale – Exemption) Order 1980) SI 1980/1924
- Access to Health Records Act
- Data Protection Act 1998
- Freedom of Information Act 2000

See *Appendix 1* at the end of this chapter for explanations of these legislation.

Resources

House of Commons Information Office: www.parliament.uk/factsheets
NMC Professional Advisory Service: www.nmc-uk.org

References

Ackerman B (2004) Statutory Framework for Practice. In: Henderson C, Macdonald S eds. *Mayes' Midwifery – a textbook for midwives.* 13th edn. Balliere Tindall, Elsevier Ltd, Edinburgh: 1142–65

Davies C, Beach A (2000) *Interpreting Professional Self-Regulation: a history of the United Kingdom Central Council for Nursing, Midwifery and Health Visiting.* Routledge, London

Department of Health (1999) *Health Act.* The Stationary Office, London

Department of Health (2002a) *Nursing and Midwifery Order 2001.* Statutory Instrument No 253. The Stationary Office, London

Department of Health (2002b) *Learning from Bristol: The Department of Health's Response to the Report of the Public Inquiry into Children's Heart Surgery at the Bristol Royal Infirmary 1984 – 1995.* Stationery Office, London

Department of Health (2004) *National Services Framework for Children, Young People and*

Maternity Services. The Stationary Office, London

Dimond B (2004) Law and the Midwife. In: Henderson C, Macdonald S eds. *Mayes' Midwifery – a textbook for midwives* 13th edn. Balliere Tindall, Elsevier Ltd, Edinburgh: 1142–65

Donnison J (1988) *Midwives and Medical Men: the struggle for the control of childbirth.* 2nd edn. Historical Publications, London

Ehrenreich B, English D (1973) *Witches, Midwives, and Nurses: a history of women healers.* Feminist Press, New York

Ehrenreich B, English D (1979) *For Her Own Good: 150 years of the experts' advice to women.* Pluto Press, London

Halksworth G, Bale B, James C (2000) Evaluation of Supervision of Midwives. In: Kirkham M ed. *Development in the Supervision of Midwives.* Books for Midwives Press, Manchester: 2

Hannam J (2004) Smith, Zepherina Philadelphia (1836-1894), Oxford Dictionary of national Biography, Oxford University Press; http://www.oxfordddnb.com/view/article/58689 accessed 12th April 2007

Hannam J (1997) Rosalind Paget and reform before 1914, In: Maryland H, Rafferty AM eds. *Midwives Society and Childbirth – debates and controversies in the modern period.* Routledge, London: 81–101

HM Government (2007a) Safeguarding patients - The Government's response to the recommendations of the Shipman Inquiry's fifth report and to the recommendations of the Ayling, Neale and Kerr/Haslam Inquiries, CM 7015. TSO, London

HM Government (2007b) Trust, Assurance and Safety – The Regulation of Health Professionals in the 21st Century. TSO, London

ICM (2005) Definition of the Midwife, Adopted by the International Confederation of Midwives Council meeting, 19th July, 2005, Brisbane, Australia

Kirkham M (1995) History of Midwifery Supervision. In: *Super-Vision. Consensus Conference Proceedings.* Books for Midwives Press, Hale

Lewis P (2007) Self regulation: privilege and responsibility. The 9th Zepherina Veitch Lecture. *Midwives* **10**(9): 414–9

Davies ML (1978) *Maternity: letters from working women collected by the Women's Co-operative Guild.* Virago Press, London

RCM (2007) A History of the Royal College of Midwives http://www.rcm.org.uk/rcm/ pages. Accessed April 2nd 2007

NMC (Education, Registration and Registration Appeals) Rules 2004 (SI 2004/1767) The Stationary Office, Norwich, www.hmso.gov.uk

NMC (2004a) *Standards of proficiency for pre-registration midwifery education.* NMC Portland Place, Standards 03/04

NMC (2004b) *Midwives Rules and Standard.* NMC Portland Place, Standards 05/04

NMC (2004c) *Code of professional conduct: standards for conduct, performance and ethics.* NMC Portland Place, Standards 07/04

NMC (2004d) *NMC guidance: requirements for evidence of good health and good character.* www.nmc-uk.org

NMC (2006a) *Midwives and Home Birth.* 08/NMC Circular 13th March 2006

NMC (2006b) *Midwives and Exposure Prone Procedures.* 10/NMC Circular 3rd April 2006

NMC (2006c) *Standards for the preparation and practice of supervisors of midwives.* NMC Portland Place, Standards 10/06

NMC (2007a) O*wnership and Sharing of Midwifery Records.* 02/NMC Circular 3rd January 2007

NMC (2007b) *The care of babies born alive at the threshold of viability.* 03/NMC Circular 15th January 2007

Stevens R (2002) The Midwives Act 1902: an historical landmark. *Midwives* **5**(11): 370–1

Symonds A, Hunt SC (1996) *The Midwife and Society: Perspectives, Policies and Practice.* MacMillian Press, London

Towler J, Bramall J (1986) *Midwives in History and Society.* Croom Helm, London

Appendix 1: Brief overview of most commonly encountered legislation by midwives

Act	Preamble	Application to midwife's role
Notification of Births Act 1907	It is statutory duty of the practitioner attending the woman during childbirth to notify the designated public health medical officer of the birth or stillbirth within 36 hours.	The duty of notification of births usually falls on midwives for purposes of planning follow up care, census and records. An NHS number is assigned to all babies at birth since 2002, it serves as a reliable, unique identifier and provides a common link between baby's records both electronic and manual, across the NHS and partner organisations. It is the cornerstone of the move towards an electronic health record.
Births and Deaths Registration Act 1953	Under the Births and Deaths Registration Act it is the duty of the mother and father or any person having the knowledge of birth or stillbirth, or taking charge of the child, to give to the registrar information and sign the register in his/ her presence within 42 days of birth. A separate registration of Death for a baby born alive and then dies needs to take place	If there is a failure to register birth by the persons concerned, the midwife present at birth may be required to fulfil this duty. There are facilities within maternity units to register births and deaths.
Stillbirth definition Act 1992		
Congenital Disabilities (Civil Liability) Act 1976 Unfair Contract Terms Act 1977 Human Fertilisation and Embryology Act 1990	This act aims to protect unborn and children after birth against negligent or actionable wrongful acts. The person is liable for wrongful actions which have caused damage and affects their right to a normal life.	The contract for care is between midwives and parents, hence it is the parents who take action against midwives for negligent care in the first instance. However under this legislation all records need to

Brief overview of most commonly encountered legislation by midwives

Act	Preamble	Application to midwife's role
Attendance at Birth Nurses, Midwives and Health Visitors Act 1979 – section 16 Re-enacted in Article 45 of the Nursing and midwifery) Order 2001	It is a criminal offence for a person other than a registered midwife or registered medical practitioner or midwifery and medical students undertaking NMC and GMC approved education programmes to attend women in childbirth except in an emergency.	preserved for 25 years and the child has a right to pursue action up to this period. This clause protects women from inappropriate care givers and also grounds midwife's role in statute. In current climate of cost effectiveness and blurring of roles role substitution is prevented.
Data Protection Act 1984 Data Protection Act 1998	It seeks to protect confidential information held on individuals. The 1998 act was extended to cover protection of manual records. It also covers access to records. Although access can be withheld in exceptional circumstances.	This act is directly related to record keeping aspects of the midwife's role especially confidentiality, consent and access to records by clients. Midwives Rules no 9 gives guidance on accuracy and keeping of records.
Freedom of information Act 2000	This act gives rights to individual to obtain institutional information from public authorities,	Midwives work in partnership with women, hence women have access to their notes – often known as hand held notes.
Human Rights Act 1998 http://www.yourrights.org.uk/your-rights/chapters/privacy/index.shtml	The preamble describes it as 'an Act to give greater effect to rights and freedoms guaranteed under the European Convention on Human Rights' (the Convention).	Humans Rights Act places an obligation on midwives to treat all women and their families with dignity and respect irrespective of their race, culture or religious

Brief overview of most commonly encountered legislation by midwives

Act	Preamble	Application to midwife's role
The European Convention on Human Rights 2000	The Convention is divided into 'articles'. Articles 2 to 14 set out the rights that are protected by the Convention. The ones most relevant to midwives are : The Right to Privacy The Right to Know The Rights of Victims and Witnesses The Right of Free Expression The Right to Receive Equal Treatment The Rights of Immigrants The Rights of Workers The Rights of Children and Young People The Rights of the Bereaved	convictions. There are some overlaps between Data Protection Act especially on confidentiality and right to privacy and Equality act.
Equality Act 2006	Under this act the Equal Opportunities Commission, the Commission for Racial Equality and the Disability Rights Commission have been dissolved and a single body Commission for Equality and Human Rights has been established; to make provision about discrimination on grounds of religion or belief sexual orientation. Duties relating to sex and disability discrimination are imposed on	This act has wide reaching implications service provision, in terms of access to care, providing facilities for freedom of expression of religious beliefs and adapting the infrastructure to accommodate the needs of disabled. The midwives will need to build this provision in their practise, especially communication, information giving and access to

Brief overview of most commonly encountered legislation by midwives

Act	Preamble	Application to midwife's role
	Persons performing public functions under this act.	care and choices. This legislation may assist midwives in tackling employment and professional issues especially, the oppressive culture, bullying and lack of opportunities
Forced Marriage (Civil Protection) Act 2007	An Act to make provision for protecting individuals against being forced to enter into marriage without their free and full consent and for protecting individuals who have been forced to enter into marriage without such consent; and for connected purposes	This is a very sensitive issue for midwives, as the women may confide in them. The midwives have a duty of care to them. This needs to be debated and discussed by organising multiprofessional education and training and developing local policies and establishing support systems for victims.

Sources : Midwives Rules and Code of Practice 1998 UKCC and Dimond 2006 Legal aspects of midwifery , third ed. Books for midwives

CHAPTER 2

Gaining Confidence and Competence as a Midwife

Rosaline Steele

'The essence of midwifery is the assistance of women around the time of childbirth in a way that recognises that the physical, emotional and spiritual aspects of pregnancy and birth are equally important. The midwife provides competent and safe physical care without sacrificing these other aspects.'

Lesley Page, 2000

This encapsulates the core activities that midwives are involved in each day of their practice. On the surface it may appear that these activities are relatively straightforward; however, most midwives would acknowledge the complexities that are implicit in everyday practice.

To care for women effectively whilst taking into consideration the challenges of everyday practice midwives need to develop the confidence and competence to practice. What do we mean when we use the words confidence and competence?

Confidence

The Concise Oxford Dictionary (1995) offers the following definition for confidence:

A feeling of reliance or certainty. A sense of self reliance: boldness
Concise Oxford Dictionary, 1995

As a student, on entry to midwifery education and training you have a certain amount of confidence in, and reliance on, midwives in the clinical and classroom environment to educate and support you as you begin to develop the skills necessary for practice. This is an aspect of the development of confidence for practice that is very often overlooked or taken for granted. Midwives and others in the clinical and academic environment, because of their professionalism, view the support and development of students as a key part of their role. They are keen to ensure that students are well prepared and have the knowledge and skills that are essential for caring for women during pregnancy, labour and birth.

The confidence and reliance that students have in their mentors and others who educate and support them effectively aid the development of their own self confidence as practitioners. Richmond (2007), in her study on mentoring in midwifery, states that mentors who were confident in their own roles enabled students to develop the skills which were essential for practice. Finnerty et al (2006), in their wider study on the role of the mentor identified the range of support that mentors contribute to students' development and which often goes unnoticed.

Development of Self-confidence and Self-reliance

The development of self-confidence and self-reliance to make decisions about care occurs over a period of time.

Students that I have worked with (both in the clinical and academic environment) identified the contribution that the women for whom they were caring made to their knowledge and skills development and self-confidence. The students indicated that as they communicated with women in clinical practice they were able to understand better and link their theoretical knowledge to their clinical activity. They felt that the linking of theory and practice helped to build their confidence as they were able to speak more knowledgeably with their mentors and the women for whom they cared.

The students developed an emotional intelligence in relation to midwifery practice. Emotional intelligence is a term which is in regular use in management and some popular literature, and can be defined loosely as the ability to perceive and access the emotions of one's self and others. The reason for introducing the notion of emotional intelligence here is to identify the need for students and practitioners to be aware of how they can affect the environment in which they work through certain behaviours and attitudes. The development of self-awareness is essential to collaborative and cooperative working and learning.

Through self-awareness and reflection you can gain a true understanding of your ability and capability. That understanding, in my experience, contributes significantly to the development of self-confidence and self-reliance, thereby enabling you to approach practice with thoughtful confidence.

Competence

Competence refers to the ability to perform the activities, which are core to a profession, to the stated required standard. In addition, a practitioner should be able to use her knowledge appropriately in new situations of practice.

The development of competence is not a once-and-for-all activity; practitioners will need to keep their knowledge and skills contemporary in order to meet the changes and developments of clinical practice. This issue is further explored later in the chapter when continuing professional development is discussed.

Tools

The Nursing and Midwifery Council (NMC) Standards of Proficiency for pre-registration midwifery education sets out very clearly the standards necessary to enter the register as a midwife (NMC, 2004).

To enter and remain on the NMC register as a midwife requires assistance through mentorship, preceptorship, and sensitive encouragement during the transition from student to new practitioner.

Supervision, in its statutory form as well as the everyday supervision that is available in the work environment, offers the support that practitioners need to help them to develop and maintain their practice.

Professional networks are essential for all practitioners as they are often a source of formal and informal personal and professional development which is necessary if practice is to remain contemporary. Professional networks provide a range of role models for the new and experienced practitioner as well as excellent opportunities to identify individuals who can offer coaching opportunities.

Mentorship

Mentorship is an essential tool in the support and development of new practitioners. Mentoring has been defined as:

> '*A nurturing process, in which a more skilled or more experienced person, serving as a role model, teaches, sponsors, encourages, counsels and befriends a less skilled or less experienced person for the purpose of promoting the latter's personal or professional development.*'
>
> Anderson and Shannon, 1988

This definition describes what is required by student midwives as they work and learn in the clinical environment. Paglis et al (2006) indicate that there is evidence which demonstrates that the nurturing process has a positive and beneficial outcome on the mentee. Campbell and Campbell (1997) reported the positive academic performance in undergraduates who were mentored in comparison to their non-mentored colleagues. They also indicated that attrition rates were lower in those who were mentored.

In my practice as a midwife, a mentor and midwife educator, I have observed the rapid development of self-confidence and clinical competence in hesitant students when their mentors nurtured them, particularly through their first clinical placement. Students of midwifery are allocated a mentor before their placements in clinical practice. The NMC has set standards for mentors, practice teachers and teachers to support learning in practice setting (NMC, 2006). The first clinical allocation is usually challenging for both the mentee and the mentor, therefore careful preparation is needed by both.

Preparation by the Mentee

Being a mentee entails having trust and confidence in the mentor and the willingness to discuss issues openly; challenges have to be accepted and there must be a commitment to the mentoring process. Mentees take an active responsibility for their learning and development, recognising their achievements and areas for further development (Alred et al, 1998).

Developing new skills and knowledge is not without challenge, particularly as the complexity of midwifery practice becomes more evident. Benner (1984) uses Dreyfus's model of skill acquisition to describe a student's development and acquisition of a skill. The model outlines the five levels involved in the process:

- Novice
- Advanced beginner
- Competent
- Proficient
- Expert.

To successfully achieve this progression, sensitive and skilled mentorship will be needed at each level of the process.

I have observed mentors in the labour care environment who have worked skilfully and sensitively with students to build their confidence and practical skills. The outcome of their action has not only resulted in the preparation of skilled practitioners, but they were also excellent role models for other students and practising midwives.

Preparation by the Mentor

Using Anderson and Shannon's (1988) definition of mentorship as a guide, the attributes of a mentor should include the ability to motivate and encourage, and enthusiasm for the role as a mentor and for the profession of midwifery. As the mentee will need a certain amount of nurturing, the mentor must be empathic, open and a good listener. A mentor with a positive outlook could be a source of encouragement to a student who is finding adjusting to a new environment difficult.

Mentors supporting students who are working towards entry on the NMC registers have key responsibilities which are set out in the NMC Standards for mentors, practice teachers and teachers (NMC, 2006). These Standards became operational from September 2006 and should be used by all who are preparing practitioners for the NMC register by September 2007.

The attributes outlined above are implicit in the standards, but more explicitly stated are:

- Good communication skills and relationship building
- The facilitation of learning
- The skills and ability to assess the student's progress
- The ability to act as a role model for the student
- The capability to create a learning environment in which the student's learning outcomes can be achieved
- Practice in manner which enhances and elevates midwifery care
- Have a knowledge base which is contemporary
- Have the ability and confidence to contribute to the midwifery programme development.

Mentors have a clear preparation and continuing professional development plan as set out in the NMC standards for mentors, practice teachers and teachers (2006). Mentors need to demonstrate, as part of the quality assurance processes, how they have maintained their professional development.

Mentoring has a range of advantages but from the point of view of the author the most rewarding aspect is supporting and enabling a colleague entering the profession to be successful and develop the ability to offer high quality care to women.

The mentee/mentor relationship will alter as the mentee becomes more experienced and skilled; this is particularly noticeable in the transition from a student to a qualified practitioner. The newly qualified practitioner may not need the support of a mentor as described thus far but will still need guidance and support for critical reflection. This guidance and support may be provided through preceptorship.

What is Preceptorship?

Preceptorship can be described as a process that enables newly qualified practitioners, the preceptee, to have a specified, formal, supported period during which they can continue to develop their confidence to practise. An experienced practitioner will normally act as a preceptor during this period. Preceptorship is not only good practice for an organisation in ensuring that new practitioners have access to formal, planned help and guidance for an identified period, but it is a recommendation of the NMC (2006):

> *'The NMC strongly recommends that all "new registrants" have a period of preceptorship on commencing employment, this applies to those newly admitted to the NMC Register who have completed a pre registration programme in the UK for the first time, or have subsequently entered a new part of the register. New Registrants also include those newly admitted to the register from other European Economic Area States and other nation states.*

NMC, 2006

The length of a preceptorship period would be dependent on the needs of the preceptee, the employer's learning and development strategy, and the complexity of the environment in which the new practitioner will be practising. A period of between four to six months is usual; the NMC has identified a period of about four months.

The Role of Preceptor

The skills and attributes needed to be an effective preceptor are not dissimilar to those of a mentor; however, the preceptor's role is different. The preceptor is now supporting a colleague who has developed the competencies to enter the NMC register as a midwife. The knowledge and skills that the preceptee has should be respected, built on, and supported. This period of transition could be very stressful for the new practitioner.

In order to enable the student to make the transition from newly qualified practitioner to becoming a confident competent practitioner, it is essential that the preceptor has the skills and abilities as outlined below:

- Undertaken an appropriate period of preparation for the role
- Have a sound knowledge and understanding of midwifery practice
- Have highly developed communication skills
- Demonstrate clear leadership ability
- An understanding of teaching and learning and in particular how adults learn
- Demonstrable ongoing personal and professional development
- The attributes of sincerity, honesty and flexibility

- Facilitation skills
- Sensitivity to the needs of patients/clients while using contemporary models of care (NMC, 2006).

The Role of the Preceptee

The newly qualified practitioner should be proactive in the preceptorship process. Contact should be made with the identified preceptor and a plan of the way in which the relationship will work drawn up. The preceptee may want to share with the preceptor her personal development plan so that an action plan for learning and development can be agreed. The preceptee, as a registered midwife, will need to ensure that her practise is congruent with the NMC code of professional conduct, standards for conduct and performance.

The competencies and standards that midwives work by in the UK should not vary, however, different employers may require that practitioners on their staff meet particular objectives. The preceptee should ensure that the needs of the employer form part of her preceptorship programme.

Effective practitioners reflect on their practice; they seek new ways of developing the care they offer patients and clients. Reflection very often moves a practitioner away from an area of comfort and security about their practice and identifies the areas for new learning and skill development (Schön, 1991). Preceptees should use the learning generated from reflection to enable them to assess their performance and as part of the feedback and discussion with their preceptors.

Advantages of Preceptorship

To the preceptee
- Reduced stress as the practitioner develops the confidence and competence in practice
- Increased personal and professional growth
- Increased job satisfaction.

To the preceptor
- Seeing the development of confidence in new practitioners
- The esteem of being a role model and supporter for new practitioners
- Access to ongoing personal and professional development
- Less susceptibility to burn out.

To the organisation
- Improved recruitment and retention of midwives

- Improved patient/ client care
- Clinical governance compliance
- A larger number of practitioners with the skills to develop and support their colleagues
- Reduced likelihood of complaints and litigation claims from patient/ clients.

Potential Disadvantages of Preceptorship

- In an environment of staff shortages some preceptors may feel overworked
- Conflict between the preceptor and preceptee
- The cost to the organisation as the preceptee has to have dedicated learning and development time.

Fortunately, the advantage of the preceptorship process outweighs the disadvantages. In organisations with robust leadership and management structures there should be the appropriate mechanisms to ensure that the process of such an important activity is well managed and supported.

Statutory Supervision of Midwives

In addition to the obvious support that preceptorship offers, midwives are particularly fortunate to have Supervisors of Midwives (SoM) whose role is to offer support and guidance about practice.

Statutory supervision of midwives has been in place in the UK for over a hundred years (NMC, 2006). Its key purpose is to protect the public. This protection is demonstrated through the support that midwives receive with their practise and in the activity of the SoM in promoting best practise, preventing poor practise and intervening where practise is unacceptable (NMC, 2006).

All practising midwives in the UK are usually assigned a named SoM from within the local supervising authority in which they practise. The midwife and her SoM meet at least once a year to review the midwife's practise and identify and plan her training needs. The midwife also has 24-hour access to a supervisor of midwives should she need to discuss a concern arising from or related to her practise.

Supervision of midwives, if used appropriately could be seen as an excellent form of peer review of a midwife's practise. The opportunity to discuss your practise in depth with a knowledgeable colleague, who is not your manager, and identifying strengths and challenges is not a development that is afforded to many other practitioners.

As part of the education and training programme for student midwives they are allocated a SoM with whom they could discuss practise issues. This interaction with a SoM at the inception of their career in midwifery should enable the student to gain a clear understanding of the role of the SoM in supporting and enhancing midwifery care and practise.

As part of the statutory arrangements, midwives must notify their intention to practise to the Local Supervising Authority (LSA) in whose area they intend to practise or is continuing to practise (NMC, 2004). Rule 3 of the NMC (2004) *Midwives Rules and Standards* sets out the responsibility of a midwife in the notification of intention to practise.

Management in the Clinical Environment

Midwives, whether they work in private or public organisations, will also be subject to supervision of a non-statutory nature. The type of supervision being discussed here is associated with the manner in which people and organisations are managed and led. As a member of a team within an organisation the midwife would have an immediate manager to whom she reports.

The manager would normally be responsible for ensuring that members of the team have a clear understanding of the standards and rules of the organisation. McNamara (2006) states that a manager would normally oversee, guide, and evaluate the activities of immediate subordinates in the organisation.

In some organisations the manager has the role of a coach with the added responsibility of ensuring that the midwife's performance review is undertaken and the appropriate feedback is received. The midwife should work with the manager to develop her personal development plan so as to make certain that funding and learning time is made available for professional development.

Coaching

The manager — as coach — could be a complex activity unless the organisation has a culture of coaching which would make it a much more natural process (Caplan, 2003). An organisation with a culture of coaching could be what Senge (1990) describes as a learning organisation. This type of organisation is committed to team learning which is an ongoing process and not a one-off activity. The lifelong learning that Senge is describing would need to have a mechanism for enabling and supporting learning, and that process could be viewed as coaching.

What is Coaching?

Coaching has been defined as:

> *'...a process that enables learning and development to occur and thus performance to improve. To be a successful Coach requires a knowledge and understanding of process as well as the variety of styles, skills and techniques that are appropriate to the context in which the coaching takes place.'*

Parsloe, 1999

Parsloe is describing a skilled individual who understands the culture and complexity of organisations with the ability help individuals to work and learn effectively in those organisations.

A midwife who is new to a health care setting as well as to the midwifery profession may find the support of a knowledgeable clinician essential to the continuing development of her practice skills. However, the development of knowledge for practice involves more than the clinical aspect of the role. The midwife would need to develop the skills of working as part of a team and those of working alongside teams. A coach, working with the midwife or a small group of midwives could help in the development of learning how to be a successful team member.

Individuals who have to interact with fellow human beings on a personal and professional level would need to have good communication and interpersonal skills. Coaching could be an excellent way of helping an individual to develop the advanced communication and interpersonal skills that practitioners need to offer care in a complex environment.

The Canadian Nursing Association drew on the work of Fuimano (2004), Kilcher and Sketris (2003) and Nelson et al (2004), to describe some of the features of coaching in the clinical environment where practitioners use their communication skills to help patients/clients develop new self-caring skills. They also indicated that timely feed back from the coach is essential for the enhancement of skills and learning.

In a number of organisational settings individuals can choose their coach. A midwife may want to choose someone who is not her line manager but has the similar breadth and depth of experience to be her coach. The arrangement would depend on the organisation's working practices.

A midwife may choose to have a coach that is external to the organisation in which she works. This would need to be discussed with her line manager and a case made for the value that would be added to the coaching process and the organisation if that approach was used. The relationship between the coach and the individual being coached is confidential and professional, therefore there should be a feeling of security about the process. However, Caplan (2003) indicates that there are advantages to having an external coach. These include someone with ability to view the working environment from a different perspective. External coaches she states, bring to the coaching partnership experience gained from other organisations, which may be beneficial to the coaching partnership.

Having access to a coach and making good use of coaching opportunities could enable a midwife to develop the clinical and other professional skills which denotes a confident and competent practitioner; a practitioner who is a role model for others.

Role Models

Positive role modelling can be a conduit through which individuals can learn about the values of a profession, a culture or an organisation. The NMC standards on mentoring and preceptorship indicate very clearly that individuals taking on those roles must act as role models for the student and newly qualified practitioners.

What Does Being a Role Model Mean?

As a role model the midwife's practice would be such that clients, students and other colleagues would be able to learn from her. She would be a well respected member of the team and in the organisation as a whole. She would participate in the socialisation of new practitioners into the profession. As a role model she would work collaboratively with colleagues across the health services, ensuring that new practitioners understand the purpose of the collaboration.

Role models would need to be very self aware, identifying where they need help to develop specific skills to support colleagues. Their lifelong learning plan should include periods of professional and personal refreshment in order to be able to maintain the level of responsibility required of them. Midwives and other professionals who are role models use professional networks to widen their knowledge base and as a source of enrichment.

Professional Networks

Professional networks enable groups of people with similar interest to share information and offer and receive professional support. These networks may be virtual or face-to-face. Midwives are able to learn of networks of interest to them through their professional body or professional organisation.

Midwives who have keen interest in research, leadership and management, normality in childbirth, supervision of midwifery and neonatal care will find networks that offer a range of seminars and other activities. Midwives who are employed as educators can access the higher education networks as well as other education development activities.

To make the most of what the networks have to offer, midwives may want to contact members of their network during the normal working day. This would identify to them and their organisation that networking is an important part of ongoing personal and professional development and of keeping knowledge contemporary.

The support that can be derived from being part of an effective network is not easily quantified. Users of professional networks use terms such as 'liberating' and 'a source of support and energy' to describe the benefits gained from the active participation in the network.

Support

The word support is very often used to describe the caring activities of an individual or charity, the statutory obligations of an organisation, a government department, or the end user agreement with an IT company.

Support for student midwives and newly qualified midwives is more than the activities of caring individuals or organisations. The support that should be offered to the student midwife can be divided into three main areas:

- Meeting the learning needs of the student and newly qualified practitioners
- Offering appropriate guidance and help in the clinical environment
- The use of clearly structured approaches when giving feedback on personal or professional development.

Meeting Learning Needs

The learning needs of a student go far beyond the planning and operationalisation of a curriculum. The approach being suggested here is what Rogers (1983) described as 'freedom to learn'. In Rogers's model, teachers in the academic and clinical environment would be facilitators of learning, recognising that the student, although new to the subject of midwifery, would have views and ideas that could enhance practice. Those facilitating student learning may want to consider the development of individual learning plans with the student so that there is a feeling by the student that they own and are responsible for their learning. This feeling of ownership builds confidence in the student.

In discussion with newly qualified midwives the author noted that there was a sense among the group that their views as students and newly qualified practitioners did not have much weight in the clinical environment. Forrester-Jones and Hatzidimitriadou (2006), in their study of students undertaking a community care certificate, noted that where students' views were met with disinterest by the service manager they were left with a feeling of powerlessness in the work place. Forrester-Jones and Hatzidimitriadou reported that the students felt they had 'no voice' to bring about change in the work environment.

If students and newly qualified midwives feel alienated or not involved in the activities of the work environment, they will not have the freedom to learn in an environment of respect and inclusiveness, and they will certainly not feel supported.

Offering Appropriate Guidance and Help

Supervisors of midwives, midwifery lecturers, mentors and managers all have key roles in ensuring that students and newly qualified midwives receive the guidance and help that they need to feel confident to practice. Curtis et al (2003), in their research on why midwives leave the profession, identified some of the real challenges which hampered learning and development in the clinical environment. These included poor working relationships in teams, approaches which could be construed as bullying, and a lack of leadership in some instances. In such environments, getting the appropriate guidance and help to aid the development of practice would be difficult.

SoMs and managers need to ensure that the standards for education and practice are being met in the clinical environment so that it is appropriate for teaching and learning.

Structured Approaches to Feedback

Theoretical and clinical assessments are a normal experience for the student and new practitioner. It is accepted that the feedback from these process are valuable learning tools. However, the manner of the feedback can and does make a difference.

Smyth (2004), in her study of students learning about the assessment process, indicated that through ensuring that the student fully understood the purpose of formative and summative assessments they were able to use the feedback they received to aid their reflection. She also indicated that feedback which was given face-to-face had a positive impact on the student's learning. Harris and Bell (1990) indicated that marks or a short comment on an assignment has less impact on learning than the use of the assignment to open a discussion about future learning needs. Caplan (2003) points to the use of effective coaching to give feedback on performance. She states that the use of real time or immediate feedback on a piece of work can be highly valuable.

Whatever mechanism is used, feedback should be given by a skilled coach, mentor or assessor, using the process that is endorsed by the organisation. An organisation with a culture of coaching and learning should have mechanisms which are supportive of students and new practitioners.

Personal and Professional Development

The preparation and maintenance of a good quality professional portfolio is an essential activity for all professionals. A comprehensive portfolio is an important tool for chronicling professional activities and achievements (Gallo, 2006).

Midwives must demonstrate that they have undertaken the appropriate amount of continuing professional development. In an environment in which education and training budgets are fully stretched, practitioners will need to be mindful of the type of learning that they choose to aid their development.

Lifelong learning is a term that may feature in a number of human resource departments. The term is used to describe the conscious and unconscious learning which is a part of a professional's life. The conscious or planned learning should form part of a personal and professional development plan. Through the development of a plan a practitioner may become more aware of the formal and informal opportunities for learning. Reflection aids the internalisation of the outcomes of learning opportunities and could help in the development of expert knowledge. Reflection on action enhances the practitioner's expertise (Schön, 1991).

Most organisations have a strategic plan which should include the role of the staff in the improvement of patient care, changing practice and moving the service forward. Midwives should view the strategic plans alongside their own personal and professional development plans, and identify how they could align their learning needs with those of the organisation. This should offer midwives the opportunity to plan their personal development, for example interpersonal skills development, or a wider knowledge of new information technology and their uses in the NHS.

The aligning of a personal and professional development plan with the organisation's strategic plan should not be viewed as restrictive. A midwife who presents her manager with a well thought out application for a financial grant for professional development which is aligned with the organisation's objectives is demonstrating her ability to think strategically.

Midwifery education has a high work based element which is necessary for the development of clinical skills. On completion of the midwifery programme, the skills and knowledge developed are still those of a novice, so transition may lead to doubt and uncertainty. Transition in itself is not without complexity as it involves a change which may result in a move to a new practice environment. There is likely to be some psychological resistance to the change. Anxiety about the unknown may account for the perceived resistance to the move into the practitioner's role. New practitioners may be able to help themselves by identifying how they respond to and manage change and develop mechanisms which can be used to make the process a smooth one.

Activity 2

1. Reflecting on your clinical experience, record the aspects of a specific allocation where you felt you learned most.

2. Make a list of the factors that contributed to your learning and how this can be extended to all clinical areas.

3. What contribution can student midwives make to improving the clinical learning environment?

References

Anderson EM, Shannon AL (1988) Toward a conceptualization of mentoring. *Journal of Teacher Education* **39**(1): 38–42

Alred G, Garvey B, Smith R (1998) *The mentoring pocketbook*. Management pocketbooks, Hampshire: www.Pocketbook.co.uk

Benner P (1984) *From Novice to Expert: Excellence and Power in Clinical Nursing Practice*. Addison-Wesley, California

Campbell TA, Campbell DE (1997) Faculty/student mentor program: Effects on academic performance and retention. *Research in Higher Education* **38**(6): 727–42

Canadian Nursing Association (2004) *Achieving Excellence in Professional Practice-A Guide to Preceptorship and Mentoring*. Canadian Nursing Association, Ottawa

Caplan J (2003) *Coaching for the future: How smart companies use coaching and mentoring*. Chartered Institute of Personnel and Development, London

Clutterbuck R (1985) *Everybody needs a mentor*. Institute Press, London

Curtis P, Ball L, Kirkham M (2003) *Why do midwives leave?* Royal College of Midwives, London

Ellsworth J (2000) Surviving change: a survey of educational change models. Syracuse, NY, ERIC

Finnerty G, Graham L, Magnusson C, Pope R (2006) Empowering midwife mentors with adequate training and support. *British Journal of Midwifery* **14**(4): 187–90

Forrester-Jones R, Hatzidimitriadou E (2006) Learning in the real world? Exploring widening participation students views concerning the 'fit' between knowledge learnt and work practices. *Assessment and Evaluation in Higher Education* **31**(6): 611–24

Fuimano J (2004) Add coaching to your leadership repertoire (mentor's forum). *Nursing Management* **35**(1): 16–17

Gallo A (2006) Developing an A+ Professional Portfolio. *A Journal for Physical and Sports Educators* **18**(5): 30–3

Harris D, Bell C (1990) *Evaluating and assessing for learning* (revised edition). Kogan Page, London

Kilcher A, Sketris I (May, 2003) Mentoring resource book: A guide for faculty, researchers and decision makers, in Canadian Nursing Association (2004) Achieving Excellence in Professional Practice-A Guide to Preceptorship and Mentoring: Ottawa, Canadian Nursing Association

Nelson J, Apenhorst D, Carter L, Mahlum E, Schneider J (2004) Coaching for competence, in Canadian Nursing Association (2004) Achieving Excellence in Professional Practice-A Guide to Preceptorship and Mentoring. Canadian Nursing Association, Ottawa

Nursing and Midwifery Council (2004) *Standards of proficiency for pre-registration midwifery education*. Nursing and Midwifery Council, London

Nursing and Midwifery Council (2006) *Standards to Support learning and Assessment in Practice; NMC standards for mentors, practice teachers and teachers*. Nursing and Midwifery Council, London

Nursing and Midwifery Council (Circular, 21/2006) Preceptorship Guidelines. Nursing and Midwifery Council, London

Nursing and Midwifery Council (2006) *Standards for the preparation and practice of supervisor of midwives*. Nursing and Midwifery Council, London

Nursing and Midwifery Council (2004) *Midwives rules and standards*. Nursing and Midwifery Council, London

McNamara C (2006) *Typical roles of a supervisor.* www.managementhelp.org/supervise/

roles.htm. last accessed on 7th February 2006

Paglis L, Green S, Bauer T (2006) Does Advisor Mentoring Add Value? A longitudinal study of mentoring and doctorial student outcomes. *Research in Higher Education* **47**(4): 451–76

Page L (2000) Ed, The new midwifery; Science and sensitivity in Practice. Churchill Livingstone, London

Parsloe E (1999) *The Manager as Coach and Mentor* 2nd edn. Institute of Personnel and Development, London

Richmond H (2006) Mentoring in Midwifery. *Midwives* **9**(11): 434–7

Rogers C (1983) *Freedom to Learn for the 80's*. Charles E. Merrill, Ohio

Senge P (1990) *The fifth discipline: The Art and Practice of the Learning Organisation.* Random House, London

Schön D (1991) *The reflective Practitioner: How Professionals Think in Action.* Academic publishing group, Hampshire

Smyth K (2004) The benefits of students learning about critical evaluation rather than being summatively judged. *Assessment and Evaluation in Higher Education* **29**(3): 369–78

CHAPTER 3

A Career in Midwifery

Pat R Donovan

Advances in technology and opportunities in global markets have made choosing a career in the 21st century a complex process. This is because career definition is changing; there are more career options, levels of expectation from a career are rising, and the entry and exit points from careers are far more flexible and un-conventional routes are far more acceptable. The notion of a career for life no longer exists and men and women entering workforce in the 21st century expect to change their careers at least three times.

A career is seen as a person's work life, a series of jobs or positions by which money is earned. It used to be thought that a specific career was chosen for life but in the 21st century people now have successive careers or multiple careers.

Women have classically chosen careers within the caring professions such as nursing and other allied professions such as midwifery. This may have been a natural extension of their nurturing role within the family and within society. Caring professions were also traditionally seen as vocational, a calling from God. Furthermore, historically women have been excluded from careers which involved higher education. This was seen especially in the medical profession but now there is an increase in the number of female doctors entering health care systems around the world. Women doctors are expected to outnumber male doctors in the UK by 2014 (Reichenbach and Brown, 2004).

Historical Perspective

In order to see midwifery in context it is pertinent to look at what has shaped the midwifery profession over the years. The context of midwifery must be seen alongside the technological advances made in the care of women, as well as the context of the education of women.

Midwifery was seen as a historic art and an ancient calling with sculptures and references made in ancient texts (Donnison, 2004). Women have always aided other women in the birth process, indeed anecdotally it is seen as the second oldest profession. The majority of midwives tended to be women that had given birth themselves and Donnison discusses the problems that occurred when regulations in Europe insisted on midwives having borne children. Midwives tended to learn their craft by apprenticing themselves to an experienced midwife and learning from them.

One of the first known text was written by Alexandrian physician Soranus (AD 98-138), who wrote a book in Greek on the art of obstetrics and diseases of women. He advocated that midwives should have clean hands and be well manicured. This was written well before science knew of the cause of infection and is still advocated today. Unfortunately Soranus also advocated some unsafe practises, such as routine manual exploration of the uterus (Rhodes, 1995).

During the Medieval ages the only medical texts written were Latin translations of the ancient Greek and Roman texts. Women would not have learnt Latin and therefore they would not have had access to these texts. During the Medieval ages there was very little medical research; it was only during the Renaissance that physicians started to question the accuracy of the ancient medical texts and became interested in doing their own research, particularly in anatomy. Before the Renaissance very little was known about the internal anatomy of the female body (especially of the developing foetus inside the womb) because dissection had traditionally been considered taboo. However the Renaissance way of thinking encouraged physicians to break old moulds and become interested in the basic facts of life.

During the Renaissance and the Enlightenment the barber-surgeons established their own Guild. It was these barber-surgeons who would be called to medical emergencies and eventually they started to take an interest in the physiology of birth. The first men-midwives started their medical careers as anatomists and surgeons. Physicians did not become involved in birth at first, only surgeons.

The Enlightenment was a very prolific period in terms of scientific discovery, and a turning point in midwifery is the first documented use of the obstetric forceps by the Chamberlen family. These forceps were initially kept a family secret as it ensured that the Chamberlens would be called for difficult births. A short summary of the Chamberlen family can be read in '*A Short Clinical History of Midwifery*' by Philip Rhodes (1995). It is interesting that although Midwifery is in the title of this book there is little reference to midwifery as a profession. Eventually the use of forceps would become widespread. During the Enlightenment and through to the 20th century there was a general decline of the traditional midwifery profession as medical practitioners increasingly got involved in the business of childbirth which was seen as lucrative, both in monetary terms as well as prestige.

Regulation

For many centuries there was a determination to licence and somehow control the practice of midwifery. The church was responsible for licensing midwives in Britain as early as 1512. This was because midwives had a responsibility to prevent eternal 'damnation' of babies who died by performing the rite of baptism. Midwives were also required to report babies born to women out of wedlock.

The way educated society saw midwives at the time could be encapsulated in the character of Mrs Gamp in Charle's Dickens *Martin Chuzzlewit* in 1844. In 1847 male attendants advocated the use of the term 'obstetrics' as distinct from 'midwifery' as 'obstetrics' originates from Latin and as such had snobbery value.

The determination to regulate and licence midwifery was increasingly resisted by the medical profession. In 1877 women gained the right to become medical practitioners and therefore male practitioners now had women to call on to assist women in childbirth that were not midwives. During the years between 1860 and 1902 and the passage of the Midwives Act the division of labour between doctors and midwives was hotly contested (Witz, 1992). This was focused into the difference between normal and abnormal labour; normal labour required assistance and abnormal labour required intervention. Doctors wanted to ensure that midwives did not venture into the area that was seen as their domain. Witz (1992) analyses this as de-skilling of midwives and this debate continues to be on-going today (Downe, 2005).

It is interesting to note that there was a movement to get midwives aligned to the medical profession in the same way that dentists are. The Midwives Act was eventually passed in 1902 and was the result of a Private Members Bill rather than a government initiative. This brought about the demise of the 'untrained' midwife (although not fully fazed out until 1940). This ensured that midwifery would be an all-female occupation with a Roll or register of practising midwives that had to demonstrate moral character to ensure their continuance on the Roll. This continues to this day with the Lead Midwife for Education signing that all entrants to the profession are of good character.

The 1902 Act brought about the formation of the Central Midwives Board which was composed mainly of doctors. It was only in 1920 that midwife members became part of the Board, and in 1973 a midwife became the Chair. Therefore, although midwifery was at last enshrined by law it was totally controlled by doctors.

Childbirth

At this time the midwife who worked with women having their babies at home continued to be autonomous, working alone, employed by local authorities and calling for medical assistance when required. But this was not to continue; women were increasingly having their babies in hospital where the increasing technology available could be applied to the process. The inception of the NHS in 1948 ensured that care during pregnancy and childbirth was free at the point of delivery.

Several subsequent government reports (Peel, 1970; Short, 1980) also advocated the safety of hospital delivery over and above the more traditional home birth. These reports were based on statistics that 'proved' that more babies died in the home than during birth in the hospital. It was only when a social scientist (Tew, 1990) looked at the evidence for these figures that it became obvious that many obstetric interventions did not serve the women they were designed for, and this is what Tew calls the 'obstetric bluff'. Tew states that optimal conditions are 'most nearly achieved by confidence-inspiring, emotionally supportive, non-intervention midwifery, practised in an environment protected from the menace of high technology '(Tew 1990). Tew's work has laid the foundation from which others have built the more 'midwifery' model of care, which sees the focus on the woman rather than on supportive technology. This was supported by the consumer movement and culminated in the *Changing Childbirth* report (DH, 1993) which advocated choice and control for the woman. The conflict between the midwifery model of care and the biomedical model of care manifests itself in clinical settings and compromises midwifery students' clinical experience. The biomedical model of care seeks to speed the process of birth to ensure that it completes as quickly and painlessly as possible.

Choosing Midwifery as a Career

Student midwives choose midwifery for a variety of reasons either because they have had a personal experience of pregnancy and birth, either by having a child themselves or participating and helping a friend or close family members, thus contributing to making an emotional choice to be a midwife with a desire to participate and help with women's birth experiences. The influence of media, career advisors, experience in the family, friends, etc. may also assist students to make a decision to embark on a midwifery career. Williams (2006) highlights the impact of an 'epiphanic' experience, when everything 'came together' on the decision to choose a career. From Williams's study on why women chose midwifery as a career a number of themes emerged, these include:

- The inevitability of the decision
- Making a difference
- Type of midwife.

Students in the sample expressed their desire to make a difference, they had a strong sense of altruism, some of which had developed from strong parental role models. For many women the desire to become a midwife is a strong passionate drive but this drive must also be tempered by reality and students need to know the demands which will be made on them (and their families) during their course.

Amir et al (2006), in their study of 260 students, found that human relationships (63.73%) and encouragement and guidance of parents (50.49%) were the most important social drives in choosing midwifery, whereas the media played the least role in the decision to selecting midwifery as a career.

Students confirm the contribution of above factors in making their decisions to choose midwifery as a career, when asked about the reasons for their choice at selection interview. However, students without children of their own express their fascination with the whole aspect of childbirth, and express that the physiological aspects of fetal development and birth attracted them to midwifery.

Despite the personal factors contributing to making a decision, it is important for the prospective students to appreciate that midwifery is a professional undergraduate programme that requires ability to study at academic level and combines this with the demands of meeting the clinical practice requirements.

Midwifery Education

One of the stipulations to being on the midwives' Roll was that midwives had to undergo specific training. In 1902, this was of three months duration, rising to six months in 1916, one year in 1926, and two years in 1938. This was for non-nurses. Nurses who wished to undertake midwifery had shortened programmes.

Midwifery courses were organised and delivered by the hospital, with doctors undertaking the majority of the lectures. Pupil midwives were employees of the hospital, and regarded as members of the workforce. The theory practice balance was in the ratio of 1:4. Each hospital had a School of Midwifery that decided the numbers to be recruited, trained and subsequently employed in the local maternity unit. The educators and the service mangers worked together and undertook each others' roles with minimal effort and disruptions. It could be surmised that midwifery had control of its education and practice.

On transfer to higher education institutions in the 1990s, midwifery education had to adapt to the academic and higher education conventions and lose some of its strong links with practice, and in some institutions it was subsumed within larger nursing faculties and suffered from the loss of its identity. A decade later, midwifery education has re-established its position, the lead midwifery educationalists appear to have more autonomy, and the links to clinical practice have been strengthened.

Admission

The entry routes to midwifery education include shortened programme of 78 weeks for registered nurses, and an undergraduate programme of three to four years for those who demonstrate appropriate entry qualifications through the UCAS system.

Recruitment to midwifery courses is over subscribed, sometimes as many as 10 applicants per place. The average age of applicants ranges from 18 years to 45. A number of candidates already possess a degree from previous studies and it is a second career choice for many of them.

The minimal criteria for entry is set by the NMC and this comprises:

- GCSE (or equivalent) A-C grades in at least 5 subjects, which must include English, mathematics and one science.

Other alternative qualifications are acceptable and many mature students opt for an Access to Higher Education course. These courses have to be 'kite-marked' and deemed to be suitable for access for nursing and midwifery. They are run in further education colleges, on a full-time as well as part-time basis. They are run specifically for those with young children and are family friendly, starting late in the morning and finishing early enough for parents to collect their children from school.

The minimal academic level for all courses leading to a midwifery qualification (from September 2008) is degree level. Degree level is seen as:

- Scotland: 260 academic credits
- England, Wales and Northern Ireland: 300 academic credits

For midwifery courses most universities will stipulate the number of points required for admission, as well as what 'A' levels are acceptable. The point system relate to the grade of 'A' level achieved:

- A=120 points
- B=100 points
- C=80 points

It must always be remembered that these are minimal requirements. Obtaining the minimal entry requirements does not mean acceptance on the course. Prospective students may see the qualifications needed as a hurdle to overcome but they are also necessary to ensure that once students are accepted on the course they have the academic ability to succeed and pass the required assessments. Universities will not want to accept a student who finds it difficult to pass examinations as this may mean that they may not be able to pass first year examinations and then have to leave the course. Although academic requirements are important, it is essential that student midwives meet the practice standard requirements.

The universities usually have additional criteria to ensure that the most suitable candidates are selected. These include :

- Personal qualities of being able to work with people
- Demonstrate qualities of integrity, commitment and ability to cope with the demands of the course
- Experience in health care setting and gain an appreciation of the values underpinning the NHS
- Ability to balance financial commitments.

The NMC is set up by Parliament to protect the public by ensuring that nurses and midwives provide high standards of care to their patients and clients, and therefore all courses leading to a midwifery qualification within the UK have to be approved by the NMC. Following successful completion of an NMC approved programme, midwifery students are entered on the NMC register of practising midwives. This gives them the eligibility to practise midwifery in the UK and in any country within the European community as long as the language requirements of that country are met.

The NMC 'standards of proficiency for pre-registration midwifery education' (NMC, 2004) provides guidance to the institutions for developing and approval of midwifery education programmes. The publication is organised in 5 sections listed below:

Section 1: Standards of proficiency for pre–registration midwifery programmes. This section contains a comprehensive list of roles and responsibilities to support midwifery practice that a student midwife must be able to fulfil on completion of the education programme.

Section 2: Standards for the Lead Midwife for Education (LME). This standard is vital for midwifery education to remain in midwives' control; it provides guidance on appointment of the LME, development, management and delivery of education programmes and thrusts the responsibility of ensuring that the student midwives entered to the NMC register for midwives are of good health and character.

Section 3: Standards for admission to, and continued participation in pre-registration midwifery programmes. This section sets criteria on age, education requirements, health and character for entry to the midwifery programme. It also provides clear instructions when there is a period of interruption of the programme or the student wishes to transfer to a different location.

Section 4: Standards for the structure and nature of pre-registration midwifery programmes. This section gives guidance on the minimum standard of education level, this has been changed to degree level from September 2008. It stipulates the length of the programme (78 weeks for shortened programmes and 156 weeks full-time) and the time frame for completing the programme. The NMC recognises the importance of student support, theory-practice balance and establishes the status of midwifery students as supernumerary.

Section 5: Includes guidance on the principles to underpin standards of proficiency. These include:

- Demonstrate a women-centred approach to care based on partnership, which respects the individuality of the woman and her family
- Promote ethical and non-discriminatory practices
- Reflect the quality dimension of care through the setting and maintenance of appropriate standards
- Develop the concept of lifelong learning in students, encompassing key skills including communication and teamwork
- Take account of the changing nature and context of midwifery practice
- Base practice on the best available evidence (NMC, 2004).

It is imperative that these standards are met by all institutions providing midwifery education, however the institutions do have the flexibility and autonomy to add local variations to maximise the learning and teaching opportunities within the programme. In reality, every midwifery education programme is organised to maximise local resources and to meet the academic institution's requirements. For example, some courses are based on a system called problem-based learning or enquiry-based learning. These courses require a high degree of independent work and self motivation. There are less lecture type sessions. This type of course will require students to work independently, as well as in a group. Others involve learning with other professional groups such as nurses, allied health professionals, social workers and/or medical students. This enables the student midwives to have a broader viewpoint and attempts to reflect the inter-professional working that occurs within the clinical setting.

Learning in the Clinical Setting

There has been much written about developing an optimum clinical learning environment (RCM and RCOG, 2007). The NMC has developed 'standards to support learning and assessment in practice' (NMC, 2007).

Most courses include a process of reflection to assist with learning in the clinical setting. This may be done via group facilitated reflection or within a portfolio or a journal. It is difficult to plan learning opportunities in the clinical area. Courses tend to be based initially on normal midwifery, but in the clinical area, on wards, and in the community working with a midwife mentor, students will encounter women with health problems as well as those with problematic pregnancies and difficult social problems. These students will encounter these problems before being taught the corresponding theory in the classroom. By reflecting on the care that these women receive students learn about the practice of midwifery before the theory. This will enable the theory to be more relevant as it can then be related to the woman's experience.

There has been a lot of discussion concerning the gap between what is taught in the classroom, the ideal, and what happens in practice. This is known as the 'theory practice gap'. Reflection is one way of reducing this gap, enabling learning from the reality of midwifery. Therefore the clinical area is not only where students can learn the practical skills of being a midwife but also where theory can be learnt using the skills of reflection. There may be opportunity to practice some skills within a skills laboratory before 'doing it' on a real woman. This is always advisable. This may involve taking blood pressure recordings, taking of blood (venepucture), as well as more midwifery skills such as abdominal and vaginal examinations.

European Union Midwives Directive

Every student midwife is required to meet the standards of proficiency to become fit for practise and entry to the midwives register. The standards of proficiency need to comply with European Union Midwives Directive 80/155/Eec article 4. These are listed in *Box 1*.

Challenges During the Course

Midwifery education programmes require skills and the ability to study at undergraduate level, and selection to the programme needs to reflect this. However, many universities experience external imperatives imposed upon them that influences their recruitment, selection and retention policies. Midwifery courses are different in that they are longer and have theoretical

---

Box 1. European Union Directives

1. Advising of pregnant women, involving at least 100 pre-natal examinations
2. Supervision and care of at least 40 women in labour
3. Personally carry out at least 40 deliveries
4. Active participation with breech deliveries. Where this is not possible because of lack of breech deliveries, practice may be in a simulated situation
5. Performance of episiotomy and initiation into suturing.
6. Supervision and care of 40 women at risk in pregnancy, or labour or post-natal period.
7. Supervision and care (including examination) of at least 100 post-natal women and healthy new-born infants.
8. Observation and care of the new-born requiring special care including those born pre-term, post-term, underweight or ill.
9. Care of women with pathological conditions in the fields of gynaecology and obstetrics
10. Initiation into care in the field of medicine and surgery.

(Source: European Union Directives 89/594/EEC)

---

and clinical components. Many student midwives struggle to complete their theoretical assignment whilst on clinical experience, and this places an additional demand. During their course students will be challenged and stretched. Students will come across many stressors, aspects that cause stress, these can be seen in *Figure 1*.

Only a few of these relate to academic studies. In my experience, changes to personal relationships and the financial hardship are the two most common factors that upset the equilibrium of coping during the course. One factor that will ameliorate these stressors is to be able to talk over feelings. This may be to a partner or a friend. However much a family may wish to support students, they also will find the course causing them stress and a change in lifestyle. Therefore it is vital to keep the channels of communication open in the home. Sometimes nothing can be done about these stressors but acknowledging them helps deal with their emotional consequences.

There are also practical issues that can be done, such as taking young children to nurseries on university sites for students' children and the availability of hardship funds. Students should never suffer alone. The universities have a number of different support systems available for students and this includes support from study skills centres, a personal tutor,

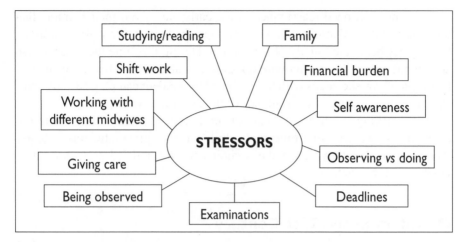

Figure 1. Stressors that a student midwife will encounter during her training.

the course tutor, clinical mentors, peers, and welfare officers for academic studies and personal difficulties.

The personal tutor/advisor who adopts a wider pastoral role are often useful sounding boards to explore solutions to what may seem insurmountable problems.

Working with Midwives

All courses have assessments related to the practice component of the programme. Students will be assigned a midwife mentor when in the clinical area. This midwife is responsible for ensuring that they learn the skills appropriate for that placement and year of the course. This midwife also has a prime responsibility for the women and families in her care. This assessment is normally carried out by mentors and also often by the midwives that students work with.

Clinical assessments require midwives to watch students as they carry out care to ensure that the appropriate care is given to women and their babies. This may cause frustrations and stress amongst midwives at having to take additional roles, especially if there are staffing problems, and students may be seen as an extra responsibility. This can be an area of conflict which students will come across and will need to report to link tutors and managers of the unit.

The clinical area can engender a lot of emotion for example students may be afraid to be left alone with a woman in labour, or the student may be asked to do something that she has not done before. This certainly caused me a few sleepless nights before commencing my midwifery course as I expected labour to be much quicker than it was.

Students will need reassurance in the early days from their mentors that midwifery skills and intuition can be developed by being there with the woman, holding her hand and quietly observing her. During this time the students can absorb not only what the midwife does but can also learn what the woman is feeling and how she copes with her birth and the student can play an active part by being there for her. This is all part of the art of midwifery.

By working with a number of midwives students gain different experiences and can fine-tune their skills. It also gives students a larger repertoire so that they can make a choice when qualified as to how they would want to practice.

Midwifery in the 21st Century

What does a midwife do in this century and what is expected of her? Men can also be midwives and they are still called midwives because the term relates to the woman being cared for and not the gender of the carer. Midwife means 'with woman'.

Partnership

Partnership is the central tenet of midwifery and central to national policy (DH, 1993). Page and McCandlish (2006) state that a midwife is a 'guardian of one of life's most important events for each individual and for society as a whole'. It is a partnership with women, but other family members should not be ignored, especially the partner and other children, as well as mothers and the mother-in-laws.

Decision-making

Decisions need to be made by the woman throughout her pregnancy and the midwife gives information that assists women to make decisions that will affect her experience of the pregnancy and birth. The midwife has a role in educating the woman as to what is happening, both to her body and to how she may be feeling.

The midwife should encourage the woman and 'empower' her to take an active role in decision making and not necessarily to just comply with what is happening to her body. A pregnant woman has no 'say' as to what happens to her body during the whole process of pregnancy, but she has a right to decide what is best for her in the area of general health, choice of type of care and place of birth, and the degree of involvement she wants family members to have during birth, as well as many other factors.

The role of the midwife is to know what is a normal occurrence and what is not. The midwife needs to know the choices and options that are available and assist the woman and her partner in making the choices that are most appropriate to them.

Communication

A woman and her partner will also have to make choices concerning the care that she may receive throughout the pregnancy, labour and the early period following birth. Communication is an essential part of the midwive's role; communication in such a way that it is easy to understand.

Antenatal Testing

One area of scientific research that has impacted on the role of the midwife and offered pregnant woman specific choice is genetics. There are blood tests available that can give a risk factor for specific conditions in the baby. The most common is Downs syndrome. The midwife has to understand the whole area of risk and be able to explain it to a couple so that they understand it and can make a decision as to whether they wish the test or not. This requires complex communication skills as well as understanding the whole area of probability, which may have been covered in maths or statistic classes. Students and qualified midwives can see therefore how communication and numeracy can be an asset.

Support

It is a midwife's role to support women, physically and emotionally during the whole process of childbirth, whether it takes place in a home or hospital environment. She is the most senior person present at the majority of births, and therefore needs to be able to make prompt decisions, at sometimes stressful times. Not all births go as planned and in some hospitals in the UK over 20% of births are by Caesarean section.

Multidisciplinary Working

Midwives need to care for women who have undergone Caesarean sections and therefore general nursing skills are also required. These involve general hygiene skills, care of intravenous and blood transfusions, and use of complex technology. This is seen as the science of midwifery. One of the competencies stated by the NMC is to 'demonstrate effective working across professional boundaries' (NMC, 2002). Student midwives will work with many other professionals, especially doctors. There may be some classes that are taken with medical students, physiotherapy students and student nurses, so that there is an appreciation of the role each of these groups play within the health service as well as with a parturient woman.

Career Opportunities

There are many career opportunities available on completion of a midwifery course and registration as a midwife in the UK. Midwives may decide to continue within the clinical area, get involved with management, or proceed into education. These are all open to all midwives regardless of whichever course they have undertaken. Most career structures require consolidation following qualification, therefore on completion of the course midwives have an opportunity to practise in local hospitals, normally in the ones that they have had clinical experience during their programme. Midwives can undertake specialist roles which include antenatal screening co-ordinator, counsellor, fetal medicine, public health, examination of the newborn, ultrasound scanning.

Although all midwives undertake 'mentorship' courses enabling them to support and mentor students, some decide to engage further in education and there are specific NMC registered courses that facilitate NMC recognition as a midwife teacher. A more recent role is one of consultant midwife; this is an expert midwife who maintains their links with clinical practice and yet are involved in education.

Some midwives may wish to work outside the NHS and join established private practices/partnerships and work as independent midwives, or set themselves up in their own practice.

Whatever midwives wish to do following their initial qualification they must keep up-to-date with the knowledge base of their profession and there are many professional development courses available from universities as well as courses run within NHS Trusts.

Midwives can further their own academic study to Masters level and beyond in Midwifery or subjects allied to midwifery, such as public health, nutrition, and physiology.

Activity 3

1. Write an account of what drew you to midwifery. Reflect on your high and low experiences.

2. If you could pass one message to those joining the profession what would it be?

Resources

http://www.ukstudentlife.com
http://alec.co.uk/cvtips
http://www.rcm.org.uk
http://www.birthchoiceuk.com

References

Amir Ali Akbari S, Arfaie K, Ahmady M, Alavi Majd H (2006) Social factors in choosing midwifery as a career in medical university students of Tehran. *Faculty of Nursing Midwifery Quarterly* **16**(52): 3, ISSN: 1605 8941

Department of Health (1993) *Changing Childbirth*, Part 1 (report of the Expert Maternity Group). HMSO, London

Donnison J (2004) A History of the Profession in the UK. In: Henderson C, MacDonald S eds. *Mayes' Midwifery: A Textbook for Midwives*. Balliere Tindall, Edinburgh: 1071–99

Downe S (ed) (2004) *Normal Childbirth: Evidence and Debate*. Churchill Livingstone, Edinburgh

Nicholls L, Webb C (2006) What makes a good midwife? An integrative review of methodologically diverse research. *Journal of Advanced Nursing*

NMC (2002) *Requirements for pre-registration midwifery programmes*. NMC, London

NMC (2004) *Standards of proficiency for pre-registration midwifery education*. NMC, London

NMC (2006) *Standards to support learning and assessment in practice*. NMC, London

Page L, McCandlish R (2006) *The New Midwifery* 2nd edn. Churchill Livingstone Elsevier, Philadelphia

Reichenbach L, Brown H (2004) Gender and academic medicine: impacts on the health workforce. *British Medical Journal* **329:** 792–5

Tew M (1992) *Safer Childbirth? A critical history of Maternity care*. Chapman & Hall, London

Williams J (2006) Why women choose midwifery: a narrative analysis of motivations and understandings in a group of first-year student midwives. *Evidence Based Midwifery* **4**(2): 46–52

Witz A (1992) *Professions and Patriarchy*. Routledge, London

CHAPTER 4

A Student Midwife's Experiences in the 21st Century

Lisa McTavish

When I first began to think about what I wanted to do with my life I was instantly drawn to a career in the caring professions. My grandmother had been a nurse, and my mother had followed in her footsteps into mental health nursing, so it seemed a natural progression to continue in the 'family business'. After a sudden decision to leave school after gaining the appropriate entry qualifications for nursing, however being too young to actually apply for the course, I was offered a job in a school for children with special needs. At this time I was still unsure which of the caring professions I was most drawn towards but after a year of working in this field I decided that Learning Disability Nursing was for me. I gained a place on a course on my first application and began my nurse training in Glasgow in 1991. I did not for a second expect that, during training for that career, I would find my real passion in life: midwifery.

The realisation that what I really wanted to do in life was to become a midwife happened in 1992 , half way through my nursing training. During our second year of training we were required to complete a public health module, including compulsory placements with health visitors, school nurses and within maternity services. Almost everyone on my course, especially the male students, were dreading the upcoming maternity placement. Having made it through over a year of general nursing placements we had already heard all the stories of the 'madwives' we would encounter on placement. Already, as learning disability nursing students we were seen as somewhat 'outsiders' by the general nursing students, however, even to us, midwives were a different species all together. As a class we were not even sure how you went about becoming a midwife, never mind what the job entailed except for delivering babies. At college we had very little preparation for our maternity placement other than a childbirth video from the 1970s so we were unaware of what we would encounter.

Being only 18 at the time, having no children of my own and no real personal contact with pregnant mothers or babies, I had no concept of what to expect, except, that I did not expect to enjoy it. I was therefore amazed to discover that not only did I enjoy it — I loved it. I found the whole process of pregnancy and birth fascinating and loved spending time supporting women, both during their pregnancy and the first few days of motherhood.

Considering the Options

I had never really thought about pregnancy and birth in any way before this experience. I began to read whatever I could find on fetal development and the process of labour and birth, and I became increasingly fascinated by the subject. I really respected the bond that the midwives seemed to have with the women and their families. My experiences of nursing at that point was that nurses were skilled at doing things 'to' people, however midwifery seemed to be much more about midwives working with women to provide the best support they could. I knew then that my real passion was midwifery. However, the option to change courses was not really feasible at that time, as direct entry midwifery was just re-emerging in Scotland, so I continued on with my chosen career.

After qualification I worked as a staff nurse for 10 years and put midwifery to the back of my mind. It was not until two separate events that midwifery came to the forefront again.

First, due to new governmental policies brought about by the *The Same As You?* report (Scottish Executive, 2000) document, there was a chance of a major change in my working life. At the time I was working in a residential learning disability unit within the person-centred planning team. The new policies were bringing about the closure of residential units for people with learning disabilities so I was working with our clients and their families to find them new accommodation and support staff that suited their own needs and wants. Although I would not be at risk of losing my job, I would be redeployed to a different post so my future was uncertain.

Second, a friend, who knew of my interest in pregnancy and birth, bought me a book that she thought I might like; the book was *Baby Catcher* by Peggy Vincent (2002). That first midwifery book re-ignited my passion and I began to read everything I could on the subject. My bookshelves began to bulge with books related to pregnancy and birth and I watched every related TV programme that I could find.

I knew what I wanted from midwifery. I wanted to support women to have the pregnancy and birth that they wanted, to empower women to believe in their own bodies' abilities to birth their babies. I did not want to be what in my mind equated to an obstetric nurse, and I worried that this was what midwifery had become. Recent research by Kirkham et al (2006) has summed up my feelings at the time about the type of midwifery care I wanted to provide to women. Kirkham et al (2006) describe how working midwives want to provide care that enables women and their families to enjoy their pregnancy, to give them a good experience, and to give them the experience that they want to have. I felt that it was important for women to be given the support they need to stand up to modern maternity services and to fight for the pregnancy and birth that they want rather than to fit into existing policies and procedures.

To reassure myself that this was possible I spent some time with my local community midwives and, on their suggestion, our local independent midwife. Between them they reassured me that midwifery was what you make it, that I could mould myself into the kind of midwife I hoped I could become.

With all this in mind, and after a lot of discussions with friends and family, I decided to go ahead and apply for the course.

Application and Entry Process

The Royal College of Midwives (2006) lists the qualifications required to enter the diploma course in midwifery as GCSE (or equivalent) A–C grades in at least five subjects, which include English, Maths and one science subject. They also state alternative entry methods such as Access to Higher Education courses and NVQ level 3 qualifications. Entry to the degree course will also require candidates to have gained a minimum of two A-level qualifications or equivalent.

Different parts of the country have differing organisations who manage nursing and midwifery applications, so being in Scotland I applied for my course through Centralised Applications for Nursing and Midwifery Training House (CATCH) rather than through the English equivalent of Universities and Colleges Admission Services (UCAS).

I made my first application at the end of 2003. Rather arrogantly I expected that I would have no problems at all with gaining a place on the course; after all I was already a nurse with 10 years of experience and lots of professional learning under my belt. When I filled in my application I wrote a basic personal statement and sent it off, fully expecting a date for my interview to arrive within a few weeks. What did arrive a few weeks later however was a brief letter, thanking me for my application but explaining that I had not been selected for interview at this time. I was shocked and embarrassed at my assumption that it would be an easy, trouble-free process

— I had never imagined that my application might be rejected.

The system of application in Scotland means that an application will only be considered by one University at a time and then passed to their next choice, with an applicant being able to state up to four choices of institution in order of preference. Being so sure of the success of my application I had only stated a first choice university, so I needed to start the whole process all over again. It was only at this time that I became aware of the great demand for places on midwifery courses throughout the UK with some institutions receiving several hundred applications for around 30 available places per intake. It was only now that I realised how privileged I would be to receive an interview, regardless of the outcome, so I decided to do my utmost to ensure I received an interview this time and a chance to prove myself worthy of a place.

I began to research more into the application process and discovered that, although I had the basic entry requirements for the course, most universities preferred their applicants to demonstrate periods of study within a few years prior to their application. I realised how important it is for applicants to prove their ability to study to a certain level before commencing the course as, although academic assessment on the course begins at Level One, it does still require a level of study that may be difficult to someone without recent exposure to education. Phillips and Bharj (1996) discuss the selection process for midwifery courses and suggest that, although it is important for universities to select students with the motivation and desire to care for women and their families, it is equally important that selected students are able to demonstrate the academic ability to manage the breadth and depth of studies at undergraduate level.

Preparation

I chose to study Human Biology with the Open University to enhance my knowledge in the biological sciences to strengthen my application and also to assist me with the midwifery course content if I did succeed in gaining a place on the course.

Around this time I also stumbled upon what was to become my lifeline, both throughout the application process and into the course itself. The *Student Midwives Sanctuary* (www.studentmidwives.co.uk) is an internet discussion board catering to people going through the application process, to present students and to qualified midwives. Through this board I could discuss applications and exchange ideas with fellow applicants. Through further searching through the internet I found that there is a lot of information available to prospective students and present students alike. The RCM has its own student discussion group (www.health.groups.yahoo.com/group/RCM_ student_midwives/), as does the Nursing and Midwifery Council (www.

nmc-uk.org/aArticle.aspx?ArticleID=2100).

In October 2004 I completed my next application, accompanied by a revised personal statement, and selected a different university as my first choice. Unlike the first time, for this application I researched several potential institutions and attended open days at my two top choices. At these open days I had the chance to speak to lecturers as well as existing students. For me there were no real differences between the two options, both came with good and bad points. In the end I picked my first choice through pure instinct, choosing the university that I felt more comfortable on the day.

I did not hear any response to my application for several months and was beginning to lose heart when, in early January, I was thrilled to receive a letter inviting me for interview in April 2005.

With a few months to prepare myself I read up on everything midwifery related. I was aware that one of the criteria for selection of student midwives at a variety of universities was an awareness of current issues in the profession as well as an understanding of the role of the midwife. Therefore on the advice of current students I subscribed to midwifery journals and read them cover to cover, even if a lot of the content was way too advanced for my knowledge at the time.

Finally the interview date arrived and, after fighting though my nerves, everything seemed to go well; the interview panel advised that it may take several weeks to make a decision. Eventually I was thrilled to be offered a place to start the course in September 2005.

Compromises and Sacrifices

Having completed my first year and just started my second, there have been times when I have questioned my desire to stay on the course. Being a student midwife is hard work, both academically and personally. The work of a midwife requires you to become emotionally involved with people experiencing some of the best and the worst times of their lives. As a student midwife you can often find yourself more emotionally affected by these experiences than more experienced staff. During the course you will develop your own coping strategies, with each student reacting differently to different situations. Hunter (2001) describes the emotional minefield of midwifery work and the different coping strategies that midwives adopt, from 'acting' techniques to emotional withdrawal.

Being a full-time student can be tiring, with full days of lectures followed by nights of studying, researching and completing assessments. Couple that with periods of full time hours on placement working hard to gain experience alongside busy working midwives whilst continuing to meet the academic expectations of university can be physically and mentally exhausting. In my experience most of our essays and assignments for university are due to be submitted at the end of clinical placement blocks which means you are often working full time hours as well as studying at home; at times like this it can feel like you need to put the rest of your life on hold for three years, sacrificing time with friends and family to make midwifery your main priority.

Before starting my course I had explained to family and friends that I would have to be fully committed to midwifery for a while and would not be as available as I had been previously. Despite this, I often find myself having to explain why I am not available, especially if I am not actually on a shift or at university, but because I have to get an essay finished or spend some time researching topics for a placement. Through this experience you learn vital student 'survival' skills, how to negotiate with everyone — about everything — how to prioritise the relationships in your life and how to try and avoid anyone feeling 'left out'. Students with children have a more difficult time when they have to prioritise midwifery over their mother-child relationships. Goldman (1999) describes her relationship with her son during the transition from full-time mother to full-time student:

> *'...for three years I was a full time mother, but that title is only a description of my relationship to one individual. I am still his mother, and I am still his mother full-time, but now I am doing other things as well, I see less of him than I used to, and I resent the way that the vile phrase 'quality time' comes to mind'.*

Goldman, 1999

I have been lucky in that I do not have children of my own and I have a very understanding partner so I can attend university and work shifts without having to worry about organising my home life too much. However I know that other students with greater commitments can at times find it very hard trying to juggle child care or part time jobs, especially when university timetables get changed at short notice or a placement off-duty is not available until a few days before we are due to start the placement.

Being able to effectively manage your time is important to help you minimise the effect that the course has on the rest of your life. Being organised and able to prioritise is essential. Being able to plan studying around placement or university, as well as home life obligations, can be a difficult skill to master and one that I am not sure any of us ever really get to grips with.

Being a student midwife can mean that at times you need to totally envelope yourself in midwifery and put the rest of your life on hold. Saying that, you do still need to make time for yourself and there is always the opportunity to switch off and forget about it all, especially when you know all your academic work is done and you have a few days off from placement — if only for a short while.

Highs and Lows

Each university structures its courses slightly differently. Some have a mix of both clinical and university days within the same week, and some courses work on a block of time in each area (for example six weeks of university followed by six weeks of placement).

Regardless of how it is structured, at times the course can be a complete rollercoaster of emotions. One minute you are on top of the world and the next you are verging on despair.

During placement blocks it can be difficult to mix trying to perform well as a student, being knowledgeable about the clinical area, forming relationships with mentors and trying to learn new skills and procedures. University blocks can be less intense with the focus being strictly on the academic side of the course. However, the pressure to perform well academically can be just as stressful, with lectures, presentations and problem/enquiry-based learning to contend with.

The majority of my highs and lows however have been whilst on placement; the highs being, thankfully, much more frequent than the lows. Some of my major highs have to be things that I know will sound trivial to others. For example, the first time I did an abdominal examination and knew what I was feeling; the first time someone asked me a question that I could confidently answer; the first time I assisted with the birth of a baby.

One of my best days was also one of my most hectic. I was on placement on labour ward which was very busy, with all the rooms full and a sitting room full of women in labour to be assessed. No one had a break all day and we all worked non-stop from the beginning to the end of the shift. It was only after it was over and we were having a well earned cup of tea in the break room that my mentor asked if I had realised that apart from confirming a few things with her I had not actually seen her all day but had got on with it on my own. That was the day that I realised that I could do this job, that one day I would be a midwife and that maybe I did know more than I thought I did. I definitely left the hospital on a high that day.

Most days have a high of some sort. A simple '*thank you*' from a woman or her family means a lot and can turn a bad day into a great day. Sometimes just getting through the day without anything going wrong can be a major high point.

Expectations

Kirkham et al (2006) consider the highs and lows of midwifery work, and one of the main reasons they found for midwives leaving the profession, especially newly qualified midwives, was the difference between the expectations of midwifery and the realities of actually working within 'the system'. The fear of the job not meeting up to my expectations once qualified has niggled in the back of my mind on more than one occasion. Many midwives in the clinical area appear to be disillusioned with their career choice. However I stick to the decision that I made way back before applying for the course that midwifery is what you make it and that I will, in time, be the midwife I want to be

Luckily the lows have so far been quite infrequent for me. Starting in a new area is always difficult, mostly due to, I think, fear of the unknown. You will ask yourself the questions: *'Will my mentor like me?'*, *'Will I like her?'*, *'Will I make a complete fool of myself?'*, *'Will the women realise I am new to all this?'*

However, even in an area where you feel comfortable there can still be very low times. Some days everything just seems to go wrong and you feel like a complete failure. Just when you think you have picked up certain skills (for example performing vaginal examinations or completing documentation) you will get something wrong that you were confident was right and you feel like everything you have learned has been lost. Midwives will tell you time after time that even midwives with years of experience sometimes get things wrong, but that does not seem to matter; you are the one who got it wrong and you feel like the most incompetent student in the world. It is at times like these that being able to share your experiences with other students really helps you to gain perspective on things. Members of my cohort are always available to listen to tales of good and bad days and can often sympathise having gone through the same thing themselves. My university lecturers are also always available, in person or via e-mail, to help me to reflect and learn from these experiences.

Pregnancy and birth is not always a happy time and there will be days where you are involved with women hearing bad news or going through pregnancy losses. Supporting women and their partners and families through these sad times can be difficult but it is important to keep a balance between remaining competent and professional and allowing yourself to show your emotions. Hunter (2004) describes the value of being able to share experiences both good and bad with like-minded colleagues:

'...expressing emotion and sharing feelings with others is immensely valuable, both for enhancing relationships and also for developing a type of practice that is open-hearted and genuine.'

Hunter, 2004

I have found that no one expects you to be emotionless, and I have always felt supported at these times by not only my mentor but all the staff. Everyone feels low when these circumstances occur, but the support from your colleagues helps you to reflect and take what you can from the experience.

The Mentors

The NMC acknowledges the contribution of mentors to the education of nurses and midwives, and has developed national standards for preparation of mentors (NMC, 2006). Mentors can make your times on placement a profoundly positive or negative experience. The majority of mentors I have been allocated to have been fabulous, they are the midwives who love to share their knowledge with students and to enable them to grow and develop into practising midwives. Having a student can be hard work for a mentor. They not only have to ensure they keep their own knowledge up-to-date at all times, but they must also be aware of university assessment policies, documents and assessment procedures. Working as a mentor does not excuse qualified staff from their 'normal' responsibilities, so having a student to mentor can be a physically and mentally exhausting time for qualified midwives. Mentoring itself is not as easy as just teaching clinical skills.

It is not surprising that at times I have stopped myself from asking my mentor questions because I have thought that I have already quizzed her enough that day and that it must get a bit exhausting having to continually explain their decisions and practice. Most mentors however really do not mind explaining themselves to students as it helps them to think about their own practice. Mentors have said that it is sometimes only when they are explaining themselves to students that they stop to think about their practice and why they do what they do. They also find it useful to have students who are maybe more aware of up-to-date research than they are, and I often find that my mentors ask me just as many questions as I ask them.

Almost all qualified midwives take on the mentorship role to student midwives. However, becoming a good mentor is a skill not all achieve. It would not be truthful to portray all midwives as good mentors. For various reasons some mentors may not be as good as others; I have came across a few midwives who honestly state that they do not like mentoring students, some say because they do not feel competent enough in their own practice (possibly because they are newly qualified or new to that particular area), whilst others say that they find it too stressful, too time consuming or just too much hard work to have a student with them all the time.

The support that mentors receive from the universities and the training they receive to become a mentor must also have an effect on their willingness to mentor. Finnerty et al (2006) state that:

> *'All mentors require appropriate practical and theoretical training for the role. Support systems for the [student/mentor] pairs (micro) and within the institutional context (macro) need to be explicit and sustainable.'*
>
> Finnerty et al, 2006

I have often found that the extra time and effort that mentors need to provide an effective learning environment for students is overlooked by managers, and that mentors are often still expected to provide care to women with the most complex needs whilst teaching their student to a high standard. Perhaps if mentors were given more support there would be a higher quality of mentors available for us students to learn from.

All mentors take different approaches to how they mentor students. Some will want you to accompany them at all times and to supervise everything you do. Others will supervise you until they feel that you are competent and will let you work independently with their support when needed. Some will throw you in at the deep end to see how you cope, unobtrusively observing you and ready to come to your rescue if and when you need them.

I was lucky to experience a fantastic mentor on one of my labour ward experiences. She seemed to excel at teaching and went out of her way to ensure that her students not only enjoyed their placement and learned something while they were there, but she also tried to ensure they gained the best clinical experience possible. She not only enjoyed teaching students but she seemed to really enjoy learning from them at the same time. I will always remember her teaching style and hope to someday model my mentoring skills on hers.

The Women

The mothers you will be looking after are pivotal to student midwives' experiences in clinical placement. The policy in the UK places women at the centre of maternity services (Osbourne et al, 2007).

The women and their families are, of course, the centre of midwifery, after all there would be no midwives without mothers. So far I have not had any negative responses with the women that I have supported during my course.

In my experience women seem supportive of midwifery students and understand that we are there to learn and might not always get everything right. I think it helps that my mentors have always explained to women when we first meet them that I am her student and that I will be providing the majority of her care but that she will always be there to support/assist both of us if needed. I am always in awe of women who allow us, as students to 'practice' on them at one of the most important times of their lives. In the labour wards I have often found women want to know how many babies you have caught — not because they are worried that you are inexperienced — but because they want to know what 'number' their baby will be and are excited that they can help you get on in your training. I have even experienced women becoming disappointed when they have had an assisted delivery because you, as the student, has missed out on catching their baby.

The midwifery I have experienced so far has been generally a very happy, privileged vocation. It is all about women, being there for them, giving them the information and support to make choices. Part of being with them is accepting who they are and respecting their uniqueness. Women do not need a robot, they need another human being whom they can trust and rely upon. As student midwives we can only nurture the women if we are nurtured by our peers and midwives who share their knowledge and expertise. As student midwives we want to be able listen to women, cry with them, pass them tissues, make them a cup of tea, and tenderly wrap their babies for them and give them the assurance that being a midwife means being with the women.

One of the big highs of this course is when a women or her family makes a point of thanking you for supporting them through their pregnancy, labour and birth. Knowing that you have actually made a difference to someone experience is a great privilege and definitely the best part of the job.

Activity 4

1. Lisa has given you her reasons for becoming a midwife. Can you list three reasons that attracted you to midwifery?

2. Describe a positive and a negative experience you have encountered that has had an impact on your practise.

References

Finnerty G, Graham L, Magnusson C, Pope R (2006) Empowering midwife mentors with adequate training and support. *British Journal of Midwifery* **14**(4): 187–90

Goldman F (1999) Transition: becoming a student midwife. *British Journal of Midwifery* **7**(3): 140

Hunter B (2004) The importance of emotional intelligence. *British Journal of Midwifery* **12**(10): 604–6

Hunter B (2001) Emotion work in midwifery: A review of current knowledge. *Journal of Advanced Nursing* **34**(4): 436–44

Kirkham M, Morgan RK, Davies C (2006) *Why Do Midwives Stay?* RCM, London

Kirkham M, Ball L, Curtis P (2002) *Why Do Midwives Leave?* RCM, London

NMC (2006) *Standards to Support Learning and Assessment in Practice.* NMC, London

Osbourne A, et al (2007) *Statutory Supervision of Midwives: A resource for midwives and mothers.* Quay Books, London

Phillips M, Bharj K (1996) Selection: a question of fit for purpose. *British Journal of Midwifery* **4**(9): 475–8

RCM (2006) *Midwifery as a Career: Your Opportunity to Make a Contribution to the Health of Mothers and Babies.* RCM, London

Scottish Executive (2000) *The Same as You? A review of services for people with learning disabilities.* Scottish Executive, Edinburgh

Vincent P (2002) *Baby Catcher; Chronicles of a Modern Midwife.* Scribner, New York

CHAPTER 5

The Paradox of Normal Childbirth: A 21st Century Dialogue

Jane Walker

Normal: *common; regular; natural; ordinary; usual; typical*
Paradox: *contrary to opinions; contrary to common notions*
Synonym for Paradox: *Riddle — anything ambiguous or puzzling*
(Webster, 1999)

The paradox of normal childbirth is a concept that has created debate amongst midwives, obstetricians, consumers, policy makers and economists, with each group having its own premise about what is normal.

When I was first thinking about my approach to this chapter I rapidly became aware that the scale and scope of the brief was daunting. Aspects for consideration range from the philosophical and biological to concepts of power and control, the structure of modern health care services and the spectre of litigation. The sociology and psychology of birth vies with statistics and epidemiology, and so the list seems endless. Somewhere in all this is the midwife and the future midwife who needs to find her or his own way. Throughout this chapter I aim to reflect on changes to midwifery practice and care that I have witnessed, participated in and hopefully challenged, and which have brought us to the extraordinary state of affairs where what is normal in 21st century childbirth is requiring clarification.

Different groups of people have different approaches to the notion of normal birth. For example, obstetricians tend to consider childbirth as normal retrospectively. Midwives, on the other hand, usually adopt a 'wait and see notion', assuming that all is normal unless there is a clear indication to the contrary. In other words, childbirth is a normal process until proven otherwise by manifestation of clinical signs and symptoms. Consumers tend to interpret normality as natural childbirth, and policy makers' and economists' perspectives of normality stem from process, outcomes and cost-effectiveness of care during childbirth.

What we notice in recent years is that there have been numerous attempts at defining normal birth (Beech and Downe, 2001). Indeed, conferences have been held and research undertaken on the subject. Whilst acknowledging the commonalities and differences in the normality paradigm from each of the groups, it is my intention to prioritize the exploration of the midwifery perspective. It is, after all, at the heart of our 'business'.

The discussion of normality in this chapter is underpinned by the knowledge and considerable experience of a midwife who has always held the 'with woman' element of the midwife's role as central in all day-to-day interactions with childbearing women; in clinical care, through her years as a teaching midwife, in the strategic planning of services, in the research process, in the minefield that is the 'politics' of birth, and last, but not least, in the overwhelming power of the birth experience itself.

To put this debate in context we should not forget that for many women across the world their concerns as birth approaches are not 'will I have a normal birth?', but rather 'will I and my child survive birth?' For them unfortunately maternal and infant mortality at birth is still very much a reality. Accurate international statistics for maternal death in many parts of the world are still simply not available (WHO, 2004), however a lack of medical facilities in many such places means that many women with complications (for example placenta praevia, pelvis malformations, etc) have no option but to have a 'natural' birth and hope for the best. I have witnessed this unnecessary waste of human life first hand while working in rural Africa where a non existent health service meant no recourse to emergency surgery, no blood replacement services and next-to-no antibiotics available. Therefore we should not be complacent in our debate.

Defining Normal Birth

Some dictionary definitions of 'normal' are listed at the head of this chapter which we need to explore. It is probably sensible to suggest that there are several approaches to such a definition — the physiological, statistical, obstetric, and the midwifery versions, as well as a childbearing woman's understanding of 'normal'. Perhaps in its simplest 'stripped down' reductionist version we could settle on defining normal birth as: *Spontaneous Vaginal Birth* (SVB). This definition is concise and to the point. However, this definition not only ignores anything that may happen during the labour (as long as the baby emerges spontaneously from the vagina and without assistance of forceps or ventouse), but it would also include spontaneous breech birth. Indeed Cronk (1998) argues that a spontaneous breech birth is another version of normal and should be treated as such (Cronk 1998), but this is not a generally accepted principle.

Despite these points, SVB does remain a simple direct definition. In 2002 Belinda Phipps of the National Childbirth Trust (NCT) described their organisation's attempt, in consultation with women associated with their work, to find appropriate words for normal childbirth. They favoured *Spontaneous Vaginal Birth,* but found that when they began to 'test' this term in the public arena, there was an immediate 'not acceptable' response, particularly from the media who made it quite clear that the use of the word 'vaginal' was not possible; much too explicit.

The NCT took note of this and finally settled on the term '*Straightforward Birth*'. I think this is a good term and one to which women can relate.

To avoid the possible ambiguity of *Spontaneous Vaginal Birth* as discussed above, we could go with the standard definition we all use everyday in our work — *Spontaneous Vertex Delivery* (SVD). It is, however, a term I find that women need explaining and will usually, after the explanation, say: '*Oh, you mean a normal birth*'.

I also have real difficulty with the word 'delivery' because it sounds suspiciously like a parcel, or even something the stork brings. It is a strangely passive term which disconnects it from the birth process: I, the midwife, delivers the baby and then gives her or him to you (the mother), whereas a woman actively gives birth to the baby with the assistance of the midwife, and this is part of the paradox.

Statistics and Normal Birth

When birth statistics are collected, deliveries and births are taken as two different items. The number of deliveries a unit has refers to the number of women who had their babies in the unit, and the number of births in a unit refers to the number of babies born to those women. These are of course two different numbers because the latter takes into account multiple births. For example, in 2006 the hospital I work for had 4,724 deliveries but 4,810 babies were born.

Every year hospitals in England are required (though it is not compulsory, so many do not), to submit activity data to the Department of Health. These data are known as Hospital Episode Statistics or HES data. The 'Maternity Tail' of these date inlcude information about the outcome of births and it is fully available for all to examine and it makes for fascinating reading (website: www.hesonline.nhs.uk).

At the last analysis published in 2006/2007 66% of women in England had a normal birth (SVD). Not too bad at first reading. However, that 66% includes:

- Women who may have been induced
- Women whose labours were augmented with oxytocin

- Women had an epidural or spinal anaesthesia
- Women who had used pethidine or Entonox.

When induction, epidural or spinal and episiotomy are removed from these figures, about 48% of women were classified as having had a normal birth. Does all of that constitute normal childbirth?

According to the work of Downe et al (2001), when you take out induction of labour, augmentation and epidural, only approximately 1 in 6 (17%) of women having their first baby in England, are having a 'normal' birth. Also, this may not include routine electronic fetal monitoring; if this had been included the figure for normal birth could decline to less than 10% (Beech, 2006).

On the other hand, women who present with a post-term pregnancy (but are otherwise completely well) and who proceed to a straightforward labour and birth following a dose of prostaglandin would not describe their births as anything other than 'normal'. Similarly, a woman whose labour begins spontaneously has one dose of pethidine, or uses Entonox, and continues to a straightforward labour and birth will describe herself as having had a 'normal' birth.

How does this help us think through our paradox? Should simple forms of pain relief such as TENS, Entonox, water birth, reflexology, and homoeopathy, be acceptable in our description of normal childbirth? I would say '*Yes*', otherwise we deny what women perceive as normal. On the other hand, induction of labour, systemic analgesia such as pethidine and regional anaesthesia such as epidural and spinal are interventions that may both interfere with the process of the birth and contribute to other interventions being required such as continuous electronic fetal monitoring and intravenous infusion, triggering the so-called 'cascade of intervention'. Perhaps these should not therefore be described as 'normal' births. (see NCT, RCOG, RCM Consensus statement November 2007: www.rcmnormalbirth.org.uk).

One of the statistical definitions of normal is that which occurs most frequently, or the mode (as opposed to mean — 'average', or median — the mid-point). In this case, the 66% 'normal' births previously described which include some kind of intervention, however benign, are in fact statistically the norm. If you take this argument to its logical conclusion, in those parts of the world where the Caesarean section rate has reached 60-70% (for example in Naples, Italy, and parts of Brazil), Caesarean birth has to be accepted as 'normal' childbirth.

Caesarean Sections
The 2006 birth data shows another rise of one percent in Caesarean births (national average now 23%).

The National Service Framework for Children, Young People and Maternity Services (DH, 2004: Standard 11 maternity specific) identified a government concern about the high rates of Caesarean section, and the recommendations are to facilitate normal birth wherever possible, within the bounds of safety:

'Flexible individualised services designed to fit around the needs of the woman and her baby's journey through pregnancy and motherhood, with emphasis on the needs of vulnerable and disadvantaged women.

'Women being supported and encouraged to have as normal a pregnancy and birth as possible, with medical interventions recommended to them only if they are of benefit to the woman or her baby.

'Midwifery and obstetric care being based on providing good clinical and psychological outcomes for the woman and baby, while putting equal emphasis on helping new parents prepare for parenthood.'

DH 2004: standard 11

The Framework (which is a 10 year strategy) also requires maternity care providers and Primary Care Trusts to ensure that:

- Staff actively promote midwife-led care to all women who have been appropriately assessed
- Local options for midwife-led care will include midwife-led units in the community or on a hospital site, and births at home for women who have been appropriately assessed
- All staff have up-to-date skills and knowledge to support women who choose to labour without pharmacological intervention, including the use of birthing pools, and in a position of their choice (DH, 2004: standard 4).

This is encouraging indeed and will help us to ensure that midwives in training are given the opportunities to have exposure to the kinds of experience that will prepare them for autonomous midwifery decision making.

Birth at home and births in midwifery led units (particularly so-called 'stand alone' units), allow student midwives to become confident and skilled, and do make a difference to the normal birth rates (Saunders et al 2000).

The internationally accepted definition of a midwife is:

'She [the midwife] must be able to give the necessary supervision, care and advice to a woman during pregnancy, labour and the postpartum period, to conduct deliveries on her own responsibility and to care for the newborn and the infant'.

NMC 2004

The NMC also states:

'Your practice should be based on the best available current evidence. You are accountable for your own practice and you cannot have that accountability taken from you by another registered practitioner, nor can you give that accountability to another professional'.

NMC, 2004

This autonomy and accountability are precious and we have a responsibility to be able to work effectively within this framework to the benefit of the mothers and babies in our care.

'Making It Better: For Mother and Baby' (DH, 2007) and *'Maternity Matters'* (DH, 2007) endorse the principles in the National Service Framework, putting access, choice and continuity of care as priorities for commissioners and providers and discussing the importance of maternity networks of care so that women can have access to the full range of community based and hospital care. The role of the midwife as a central person in maternity care is reflected in *'Making it Better'* and endorsed in *'Maternity Matters'*.

Midwifery Education

What are the implications of these statistics for student midwives and their education programmes? Those of you currently going through midwifery training programmes will be only too aware of the current requirements: 40 normal deliveries; 40 complicated deliveries; an unspecified number of vaginal examinations; 100 antenatal examinations; and 100 postnatal examinations of mother and baby. However I wonder how difficult you are finding it to get your 'normal' deliveries?

Reflecting this dilemma, in 2006 the NMC put out a consultation paper about future competencies that might be required for student midwives. To facilitate a response to the consultation document I brought together a group of midwives that I currently work with, some of whom are Supervisors of Midwives, and we discussed our response. The most controversial part of the document for everyone was the discussion around the '40 normal births'. It was being suggested by the NMC that because it is so difficult for students to gain experience of 'non-interfered with births' (my words), that we were being asked re-evaluate what kinds of birth can be included in the term 'normal'. It was suggested that elements of care such as induction of labour or the use of epidural should be included in the 'normal' birth tally, as long as they resulted in a spontaneous birth.

However I have met student midwives coming towards the end of their education programme who have said they have never looked after a woman in labour without an epidural. How can anyone understand either the physiological processes of normal childbirth or a woman's 'normal' response to labour, if they have never observed a labour that proceeds without an epidural?

Being a midwife has at its core the knowledge of what it means to be alongside a woman as she takes the unknown journey of labour; to be able to recognise when her responses to the labour are out of the ordinary or when the progress of the labour is deviating from normal. The midwife has to be able to help her, reassure her, give courage and guidance, and you cannot do this if you do not recognise the normal physiological responses of labour and birth. This knowledge is especially important if the labour is occurring outside the confines of a standard hospital labour ward. In other words, concentrating solely on the final outcome of the process of labour rather than the process itself is not enough.

Overemphasis on the final outcome implies, perhaps, that what happens in the pregnancy and labour is irrelevant because the end result was a 'normal' delivery. Unfortunately, that may not be the woman's recollection of the events of labour. I say unfortunately because I spend many hours as a consultant midwife listening to women's stories of feeling: *'out of control'*, 'a *lump of meat'*; *'I still have flashbacks about people shouting at me'*; *'nobody came near me for hours it seemed'*; *'I just needed to get those belts off my belly and walk about, I couldn't bear being on the bed'*. All these women had 'normal' births, yet their memories contradict that description.

Labour and birth are not just physiological events but also social and psychological ones. Jowett (1993) considers that: 'Labour is women's work and "managed" by women's minds', and Rothman (1996) describes birth as:

'Birth it seems is very much what we make of it; an ordeal, a procedure, an event, a spectacle. Birth can be medical, sexual, empowering, belittling, spiritual, humiliating, joyous, terrifying, routine – often it is all those things at once'.

Rothman, 1996

A labour can be disrupted by elements other than the physical nature of the labour, and a midwife needs to be able to understand the subtle influences on that labour so that she can support the woman with appropriate skill. These skills are not learned by only caring for women in labour who have an epidural in place. The current reduction of opportunities for student midwives to experience 'non interfered with birth' will lead, unless we are very careful, to a continuing loss of understanding of the processes of normal birth and by default the confidence and knowledge of how we work with women to progress through labour and have a normal birth. As long as obstetric labour wards are where students gain the most of their experience of birth the more likely it is that they will become, as midwives, afraid of working outside the confines of the 'managed labour' ward environment and we will run the risk of women continuing to experience unnecessary interventions in their otherwise normal labours.

Normal Physiological Birth

Perhaps the time has come to put in words a description of normal birth from a physiological and midwifery perspective:

> *'A normal birth is one that follows an uncomplicated pregnancy; with a labour that begins spontaneously somewhere between thirty seven and forty two weeks of said pregnancy, with the fetus in a longitudinal lie, vertex presenting. Mother and baby respond appropriately to the stress of labour and the woman moves about freely. Surveillance of the fetal heart rate is by intermittent auscultation...Steady progress is made.'*

You may wish to pause for a moment and think about your own present understanding of what constitutes progress in labour.

> *'As contractions gradually increase in length, strength and frequency they are combined with purposeful dilatation of the cervix and descent of the presenting part until full dilatation of the cervix is reached and the onset of second stage begins. Membranes are left to rupture spontaneously.'*

Dear student, are you absolutely clear about what constitutes a pre-labour phase, a latent phase of first stage, an active phase of first stage, a transition phase and the physiological differences between a first labour and subsequent labours? Also, go and read again about the phases of second stage: the latent phase, the active phase and the perineal phase. Let us continue:

> *'The onset of second stage may be characterized by an initial pause or spacing out of contractions (the resting phase), such a welcome break from the crazy intensity of the last hour of first stage, but as the head descends, the strong expulsive contractions begin to build until a powerful, unstoppable momentum takes hold. The woman reaches up spontaneously to find something to hold onto. She will squat down, kneel in some way or stand. The vertex is visible and continues to make descent*

until the perineum is stretching. The woman controls the stretching with short expulsive breaths; she may reach down to feel her baby's head. She does not need to be told what to do she just needs your professional observance, human encouragement and re-assurance. Second stage ends with the complete spontaneous expulsion of the baby from the vagina and the onset of respirations. There is no, or minimal, damage to the mother's perineum...Mother, baby and family begin to get to know each other.'

'Third stage — spontaneous delivery of the placenta and the control of haemorrhage occurs without incident.'

How many of these births have you observed or conducted?

Shaheeda's Story

I would like to share with you a recollection of an important moment from my own midwifery experience. All names have been changed to maintain patient confidentiality. It was in early 1982 when women in hospital almost always laboured on the bed (often for hours) and the birth itself was conducted with the woman in a recumbent or slightly semi-recumbent position (mother's feet on the midwife's hips mode), midwife gowned and masked, and with lots of very vocal instructions to 'hold your breath, chin on your chest and push'. Episiotomy rate for primigravidae was 90%.

In 1982 a young woman newly married and newly arrived in the UK presented with a full term pregnancy for care in labour. She had almost no understanding, or use of, spoken English apart from basic civilities. This was her first experience of birth, and I was to be her midwife.

Shaheeda was just 16 years old. A young Muslim girl brought up in a village in Pakistan, for whom, following cultural tradition, the onset of menstruation signalled her readiness for marriage. Her marriage had been arranged with a young man (a cousin) born and brought up in East London, whose family was from the same village. He was 19 years old and was referred to dismissively by the women who accompanied Shaheeda, as 'the boy father'. He played no part in the drama of this birth. He appeared only once to see his young wife during her labour and his visit prompted her to pull the bed sheet over her head so that she could not see or be seen by him. He was sent away.

Shaheeda was accompanied in labour by her mother-in-law and two sisters-in-law. Only one of these people spoke English, and this was a 12 year old girl called Sumi. It was reluctantly agreed by the older women that because of this (her English fluency) Sumi would be the one person who was 'allowed' to accompany Shaheeda into the birth room; it was very clear that they would all have preferred to come together.

Sumi watched her sister-in-law carefully throughout the labour and apparently completely without fear. Sumi served as translator for me and also as observer. She made little attempt to give spontaneous emotional, physical or verbal support to Shaheeda which, given her young age, was perhaps to be expected. She did, however, take a lot of interest in the proceedings, asking me questions about many aspects of labour and birth. Whenever I commented to her about how well Shaheeda was coping with it all, Sumi would simply shrug her shoulders and add 'She's always very good'. Shaheeda herself, despite her young age and, for all I knew, limited formal education, proceeded to cope with her experience of first birth with power and dignity and she gave me, as her then relatively inexperienced midwife, my first encounter with a woman's instinctive behavioural response to the powerful, spontaneous physiology of birth. She stood, rocked, moaned gently, paced, squatted and rested in an entirely instinctive manner, working in harmony with the biological directions of birth. Even when she was removed from the company of the older women into the sterile, hostile environment of the contemporary labour room, this teenager, dislocated from her own country, language, family and loved ones, coped with labour and birth with determination and strength and I had the privilege of participating in a powerful but gentle 'non-bed' birth (my first), and though I was reprimanded in no uncertain terms for this afterwards, the experience was to influence my practice profoundly forever.

The contact I have with student midwives now leads me to understand that for most of them the only time they experience a labour like that described above is if they have the opportunity to participate in a home birth or a community midwife-led birth centre facility (Walsh, 2006; Saunders et al, 2000; Walker, 1998, 2001). These opportunities are not readily available in most training circuits and students will usually have to be willing to be 'on-call' to secure this option. I advise you to make every effort to do this. Many students I have met will use their 'elective' period to try to arrange a placement that gives them the experiences many of them crave, some of them travelling many miles away from home to achieve this.

Perhaps the educational institutions should be insisting that a full range of birth environments should be available for the placement of students, rather than 'dumb down' the definition of normal birth.

Those students who are distressed at the nature of the experiences available need to develop coping mechanisms. Notice midwives who work in a way that facilitates women being active in their labours, who readily offer women the use of the pool in labour and who are regularly putting themselves forward to attend home births; seek them out, approach them, and see if they would agree to be your mentor. Consider what skills you want to acquire to help you learn how to facilitate normal birth and that may mean attending courses outside of your regular programme (with the National Childbirth Trust or the Active Birth Centre, for example).

Above all, listen to women, their hopes and expectations of birth, and afterwards their experiences of birth. Be meticulous in your learning, know everything there is to know about the three Ps: the Powers, the Passenger and the Passages. There is no substitute for knowledge.

Future Perspectives

We are entering a period of real opportunity as local Commissioners of services (PCTs and GPs) construct their strategies for the future frameworks for maternity. The options for developing and strengthening midwifery led care in antenatal and place of birth arrangements will be there. We must be ready to influence decision making and grasp the initiative. In the 'brave new world' of children's centres and community maternity centres and 'polyclinics', midwives and their students will be able to build the continuance of midwifery knowledge in the arena of normal birth. Perhaps in 10 years time the 'paradox' of normal childbirth will be assigned to history.

Activity 5

1. Write a story of your experience that has made a lasting impact on your practise and that you could share with others.

2. Write a short piece outlining your vision of midwifery.

References

Beech B (2006) Making it Real, Making it Better. *Aims Journal* **18**(1): 12, 13

DH (2004) *National Service Framework for Children, Young people and Maternity Services.* DH, London

DH (2007) *Making It Better: For Mother and Baby, Clinical case for Change.* DH, Lodon

DH (2007) *Maternity Matters: Choice, access and continuity in a safe service.* DH, London

Downe S, McCormic C, Beech BAL (2001) Labour Interventions associated with Normal Birth. *Br J Midwifery* **9:** 602–6

Downe (2001) Midwives Information and Resource Service Hot Topics Study Day Defining normal birth, evidence from the Trent Normal Birth Survey City Hospital, Birmingham 21/5/2001

Downe S (2004) Is there a future for normal birth? In: Wickham S ed. *Midwifery Best Practice2*. Elsevier (books for midwives)

Cronk M (1998) Midwifery Skills needed for Breech Birth. *Midwifery Matters* **78:**

Jowett M (1993) *Childbirth Unmasked*. Peter Wooller

NHS Maternity Statistics 2004/5, Published 2006, The information Centre, Community Statistics. www.hesonline.nhs.uk

Rothman BK, (1996) Women, Providers and Control. *Journal of Obstetric Gynecologic and Neonatal Nursing* **25**(3): reprinted in; *MIDIRS Midwifery Digest* (Dec 1996) **6**(4): 479–82

Saunders D, Boulton M, Chapple J, Ratcliffe J, Levitan J (2000) Evaluation of Edgware Birth Centre, North Thames Perinatal Public Health, January 2000

Walker J (1998) The Edgware Birth Centre: A service for women and babies at the leading edge of midwifery practice. *MIDIRS Midwifery Digest* **8**(3): 376–9

Walker J (2001) Edgware Birth Centre: What is the significance of this model of care? *MIDIRS Midwifery Digest* **11**(1): 8–12

Walsh D, Rashad A, Downe S (2004) Risk, Safety and the Study of Physiological Birth. In: Downe S ed. *Normal Birth, Evidence and Debate*. Elsevier, Oxford

Walsh D (2007) *Small is Beautiful: Lessons for Maternity Services from a Birth Centre*. Radcliffe Publishing Ltd

Walsh D (2007) *Evidence-Based Care for Normal Labour & Birth*. Routledge, London

Webster (1999) *Webster's New International Comprehensive Dictionary of the English Language*. Deluxe Encyclopedic edition. Trident Press International

World Health Organisation (2004) *Maternal Mortality in 2000*. WHO, Geneva

Recommended Further Reading

Davies E, Harrison L, Arms S (2004) *Heart and Hands: A Midwife's Guide to Pregnancy and Birth* 4th edn. Celestial Arts, California

Ancheta R, Simkin P (2005) *The Labor Progress Handbook*. 2nd edn. Blackwell Publishing, London

CHAPTER 6

Understanding Evidence-based Midwifery Practice

Tina Lavender

Evidence-based practice is well developed in obstetrics (Audit Commission, 1997) and has become the accepted norm in maternity care. The notion that the care we provide should be supported and justified by some tangible means has been driven by a number of factors, including the desire to provide optimum care, the needs of women to know the rationale for care provided, and the increasing need to defend practice in case of litigation.

Advances in technology, skills and knowledge coupled with social and environmental changes make it necessary for all practitioners to keep up-to-date and use evidence appropriately. It is no longer acceptable to practise in the way that practice has always been carried out. This means that the new generation of midwives need to be critical thinkers with enquiring minds.

Student midwives cannot rely solely on their mentors to demonstrate evidence-based practice. In preparation for being a qualified midwife, students need to use their time to question practice, explore the evidence and, if necessary, challenge the *status quo*. Students can only do this if they understand what evidence-based practice is.

What is Evidence?

The term 'evidence' is difficult to define as it means different things to different disciplines and is interpreted in various ways by individuals. In its simplest form it is the basis for belief or disbelief: *knowledge on which to base belief*. However, most often, when used in health care, 'evidence' refers to research evidence. Below are two useful definitions of research evidence.

Research is a systematic, formal rigorous and precise process employed to gain solutions to problems and/or to discover and interpret new facts and relationships. (Waltz and Bausell, 1981). It is the process of looking for a specific answer to a specific question in an organized objective reliable way (Payton, 1979).

However, within the health care system generally, and midwifery specifically, there is a dearth of evidence from which practice can be informed. As a consequence practitioners need to draw on many different forms of evidence to inform their actions, some of which are not empirical (formal). As can be seen in *Figure 1*, there are many forms of evidence that we use, consciously or unconsciously.

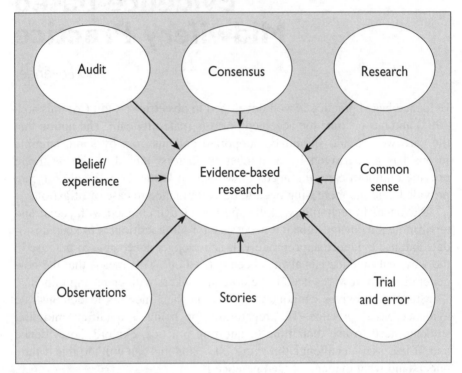

Figure 1. Sources of evidence

In many situations, empirical evidence is not required. For example, we do not need research to tell us to be kind to women, and we do not need empirical evidence to tell us that it is best to bathe a baby in warm water. In these situations we need to draw on common sense.

In other situations we just get a 'hunch' or a 'gut feeling' about a situation, and this can happen against what is perceived to be the strongest current evidence. For example, a midwife who is caring for a woman who is progressing slowly in labour may say to herself: '*I know that Mrs X's contractions are going to get stronger shortly and she is going to give birth without intervention.*' This can provide the new midwife with a difficult dilemma, especially if local guidelines dictate a particular practice, for example, the use of oxytocin to accelerate labour. The experienced midwife, however, will combine all the available evidence to provide a suitable plan of care. The midwife will know that current definitions of labour length are arbitrary and not based on any strong evidence (Lavender et al, 2005). She will therefore draw on her knowledge of the woman; how she is coping, what her wishes are, and what condition the mother and baby are in. She will allow her previous experiences to inform her actions and will draw on common sense. Her common sense, for example, will tell her that the woman should be observed. The midwife may also decide to discuss the plan of care with colleagues. Communication is an important part of the midwife's role, and seeking advice should be seen as a strength and not a weakness. Finally, the midwife will record her actions, justifying the course she has taken. Unfortunately, midwives are better at recording the rationale for a treatment or intervention than they are for deciding to do nothing but observe. This is equally important, as only the attending midwife will know what evidence she drew upon at that particular time for that particular woman.

What Evidence Counts?

A number of hierarchies of evidence have been developed to enable different research methods to be ranked according to the validity of their findings (see *Table 1*). However, 'evidence' is contentious, especially when the 'gold standard' is held to be data arising from randomised controlled trials, leading some to question the adequacy of existing hierarchies when evaluating healthcare (Evans, 2003). Most research has focused on evaluation of the effectiveness of interventions, such as magnesium sulphate for the treatment of pre-eclampsia, or external cephalic version (ECV) for the prevention of breech births.

Sackett et al's (2000) hierarchy of evidence is often utilised, but has provoked much unresolved controversy about the kind of evidence that is actually most relevant to practice; for example, controlled trials often restrict the kind of women recruited, whereas cohort studies better reflect whole populations and normal patterns of care.

Randomised Controlled Trial

Whilst the randomised controlled trial appears to be the most reliable way of testing whether an intervention improves outcome, and has received a recognised status within evidence-based care, it must be noted that the meta-analysis remains the gold standard as it takes into account the results of numerous randomised control trials.

Unfortunately, however, the randomized controlled trial fails to address women's perspectives and experiences (Oakley, 1990).

Table 1. The hierarchy of levels of evidence

1.	A	Systematic reviews/ meta-analyses
	B	Randomised controlled trials
	C	Experimental designs
2.	A	Cohort control studies
	B	Case-control studies
3.	A	Consensus conference
	B	Expert opinion
	C	Observational study
	D	Other types of study, for example interview-based, local audit)
	E	Quasy-experimental, qualitative design
4.		Personal communication

The problem with randomised controlled trials is that they produce only population-based outcomes, i.e. although the results apply to the majority, they do not allow for individual variations. Thus, the evidence drawn from them may not translate directly into the best care possible for an individual woman or reflect the skills and experiences of a specific midwife. Indeed, David Sackett and colleagues have stated that evidence-based medicine is:

'...the integration of best research evidence with clinical expertise and patient value'.

Sackett et al. 2000

When randomised controlled trial evidence is translated into formal hospital clinical guidelines, midwives, being employees of that hospital, may be held in breach of contract if they do not adhere to them. To deviate from such guidelines, midwives need to be familiar with the evidence and be able to relate findings to individual scenarios.

Randomised controlled trials, however, have in fact contributed to reducing many intrapartum interventions. Without randomised controlled trials we would still be carrying out, for example, routine perineal shaves on all labouring women (Besevi and Lavender, 2006), and routine episiotomies (Carroli and Belizan, 1999).

However, if randomised controlled trials inform guidelines that are deemed to be inappropriate for an individual woman, this can become a real issue. In such situations it is imperative that the midwife knows the strength of the evidence and is able to contextualise this evidence and relate it to the particular woman's situation, although the midwife should discuss this with colleagues. It is important to remember that, although working in the best interests of the woman, midwives, like anybody, do not always get things right. Gaining a sense of others' views can aid the decision-making process.

Qualitative Research

Until recently qualitative research was not seen as an important part of evidence and given little prominence within maternity care. As stated by Kingdon (2004):

> '...the emerging clinical governance agenda has had a positive impact on the status of qualitative research as there has been an increasing recognition that its methods of inquiry are often the only way to understand both health processes and their influence on health outcomes from the perspectives of those receiving care'.

Kingdon, 2004

In its simplest terms, qualitative research is a process that involves the collection, analysis and interpretation of data that are not easily reduced to numbers (Murphy et al, 1998). Qualitative research enables researchers to explore issues and ask questions, for example: *What aspects of maternity care are important to women? How does what is important to them vary depending on their situation?* Qualitative research can inform practice as a stand-alone piece of work or can be used in conjunction with a clinical trial.

Mavis Kirkham's (1991) seminal work exploring midwives' information-giving during labour offers an important example of a stand-alone qualitative study.

However, qualitative research alongside a randomised controlled trial is also becoming more popular. The realisation of its usefulness in interpreting trial findings has been one of the drivers of this transformation. Furthermore, according to Snowdon et al (2004):

'The use of such data alongside quantitative data represents a shift to a more holistic, integrated view in which an intervention is not seen solely in a narrow clinical focus but in a social context'.

Snowdon et al, 2004

Narrative accounting, or story-telling, is not given much status within hierarchy tables. Nevertheless, it is increasingly being used as a tool to reflect on health care and is likely to gain in strength.

Perez-Botella and Downe (2006 a,b) provide an excellent example of how story-telling techniques were used to describe and reflectively analyse the practice of directed pushing in second stage labour. The practice is endemic despite evidence from formal research that it does not benefit women and babies, and, indeed, that it may be harmful. Within this paper, the lessons from the narrative account are discussed alongside the formal evidence base and highlights the potentially dramatic impact that story-telling could have in the shaping of maternity services when constructively used as a tool to inform practice.

Assessing the Evidence

Going through all the processes to make evidence-based decisions can be time-consuming, especially if you do not have adequate skills to apply them. Additionally, despite your best efforts, you may not be able to find high-quality evidence for many of the clinical decisions you must make. However, over the last two decades there have been numerous advances in evidence processing, including the production of streamlined guides to aid critical appraisal of the literature, evidence-based abstraction services, online and other forms of electronic literature searching, growing numbers of high-quality systematic reviews, and frequently updated textbooks in paper and electronic formats. The main sources of empirical evidence are as follows:

Primary Literature
Original research papers, reporting the methods and findings of one particular study.

Systematic Reviews
An amalgamation of the findings of a number of primary studies. A systematic review is a review in which evidence is systematically identified, appraised, and summarised according to pre-defined, explicit methods. The aim of a systematic review is to integrate the findings, pool the data where appropriate, and generate 'overall' results.

Evidence-based Practice Guidelines
Guidelines which have been developed by reviewing and appraising the available evidence in a given field.

Consensus Development Reports
Reports that have been developed through formal consensus by known experts within a given field, who may draw on available evidence.

Appendix 1 at the end of this chapter details a number of useful sources of evidence in maternity care.

Finding the best evidence for a given situation needs careful thought. Many inexperienced midwives fall into the trap of finding isolated research papers and fail to systematically review all the available evidence. This can create a misleading view of the findings. For example, if you were exploring postnatal debriefing and read only one paper which showed a positive result from this practice it would be easy to be convinced that this was an effective intervention. If however you carry out a systematic review of the evidence, whereby the results of a number of studies are pooled, the findings would be inconclusive.

The quantity of research papers in a given topic area does not equate to the quality. There could be a wealth of papers, all of poor methodological quality. Alternatively, there could be only one paper of good methodological quality. Fortunately, however, systematic reviews of many of the major areas of maternity care have already been conducted. Midwives, therefore, need to understand how to access them.

Search Strategies and Techniques

It is important that midwives develop the skills to search the key bibliographic databases and other sources of evidence. You should avail yourself of the information literacy (user education) sessions provided by your university library and by NHS libraries. You can also make use of the many online tutorials and resource guides for evidence-based practice. Ebenezer (2007) provides a comprehensive list of these.

After you received training on the use of a particular resource, you should consolidate your skills as soon as possible by carrying out your own searches. The search interfaces of the major resources for evidence-based practice are designed to be intuitive and user-friendly as far as possible, but using them effectively requires some training and practice. Note that some bibliographic databases, such as Medline, are available via a variety of interfaces (such as OVID and WebSPIRS).

It is important when you carry out a search on a clinical topic that you clarify beforehand the question you are asking. For example, clinical questions may usefully be formulated using the PICO structure (Patient [Woman], Intervention, Comparison, Outcome). For more social science-based topics, SPICE (Setting, Population, Intervention, Comparison, Evaluation) may be more appropriate.

Once you have formulated your question in this way, it can readily be translated into a search query. How this is done will depend on the resource you are searching and the search functionality that is available. For good examples, see Schardt and Mayer (2004) (PICO) and Booth and Dixon-Woods (2004) (SPICE).

Many people make the mistake of assuming that bibliographic databases work in the same way as internet search engines; they type a single term or short phrase into the search box. However, information retrieval from these databases works in a different way. The bibliographic records contain (of articles, book chapters, reports) are structured into a number of different fields: author, title, journal title, publication year, abstract, publication type, and so on. Bibliographic database search functionality is much more powerful than that of internet search engines, and usually offers features such as:

- Automatic mapping from search keywords to thesaurus terms
- The ability to combine terms in a query using the 'Boolean' operators AND, OR and NOT, and with proximity operators (these specify that the terms occur together within a field, or a particular distance apart within a sentence)
- Retention of the search history, hence the ability to re-use earlier searches in new search statements
- The ability to limit searches by date, client group, country of publication or publication
- Word stem searching or truncation
- Phrase searching.

The thesaurus of a bibliographic database is a structured list of approved subject headings (preferred terms) showing the relationships between them. The ability to map to thesaurus terms is a particularly useful and significant search feature. In general, you should always carry out subject searches using thesaurus terms (also called descriptors) since you will thereby improve the precision (or specificity) of your search, and save yourself the trouble of carrying out multiple searches on synonymous keywords. These technical aspects of searching are discussed in detail by Booth and Dixon-Woods (2004.)

What is Evidence-based Practice?

Evidence-based practice is about using rather than doing research. It is therefore not expected that all midwives become active researchers, but all midwives should be evidence-based practitioners.

Evidence-based practice is aimed at improving healthcare delivery, it considers use of resources, focuses on a range of outcomes, acts as a tool for delivering education and is useful for standard setting. This range of characteristics represents the multifaceted nature of evidence-based practice, demonstrating that it is not simply about applying a piece of research into practice; instead it is about using the available evidence, in context. *Figure 2* shows the holistic nature of evidence-based practice and that evidence from experimental research alone may not always lead to evidence-based practice.

This can be related to a particular midwifery practice, for example water births; then it becomes clear that there are a number of influencing variables (see case example below and *Figure 3*).

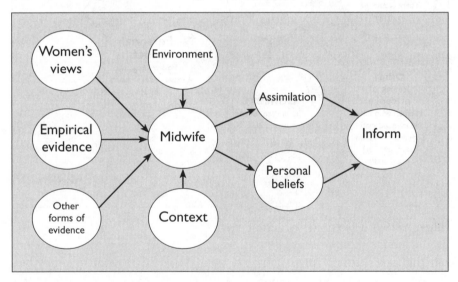

Figure 2. Influencing variables to informing practice.

Case Example: Water Birth

Caring for women during pregnancy and birth has a profoundly human element where clinical judgement is also informed by social context. It is widely acknowledged that randomised controlled trials are the best source of evidence of the effectiveness of clinical interventions (Popay and Williams, 1998; Miller and Crabtree, 2000). However, evidence of effectiveness alone does not necessarily mean an intervention will be widely implemented.

Conducting a randomised controlled trial is a pointless exercise if the results are not acceptable to women and/or midwives. In *Figure 3*, it is clear that if a woman does not wish to labour in water then the evidence is unlikely to be influential.

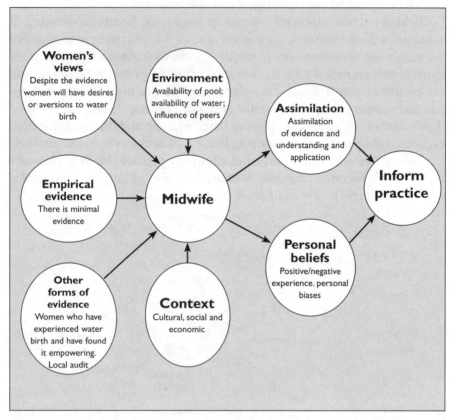

Figure 3. Water birth.

Bewley and Cockburn (2002) make reference to an ongoing powerful debate taking place in the medical and lay press regarding elective caesarean section for 'maternal request' even in normal uncomplicated pregnancies. However, as professional concerns promoting physiological birth at one end of the spectrum and caesarean section at the other are increasingly taking centre stage, there is a danger of losing sight of the fundamentally important question of how the individual women accessing contemporary maternity care actually feel about elective caesarean section in the absence of a clinical indication. Evidence-based practice must always give priority to individual women's wishes.

Therefore, although a randomised controlled trial offers answers to questions about effectiveness and safety which individuals cannot answer from the experience of individual cases (Oakley, 2000), other forms of evidence can influence whether practice changes are made.

Midwifery is more than the application of scientific rules that dictate practice. Midwifery is an art and a science and both need to be applied in practice. Breastfeeding is a prime example of this: a midwife needs to understand the physiology of breastfeeding, the empirical evidence related to successful lactation and the social influences on individual women's experiences. Therefore, as stated by Muir Gray (1997), evidence-based practice is:

'...an approach to decision making in which the clinician uses the best evidence available, in consultation with the patient [woman], to decide upon the option which suits that patient best'.

Muir Gray, 1997

Similarly, Greenhalgh (1997) states that:

'Evidence-based medicine requires you not only to read the right papers at the right time and then alter your behaviour (and, what is often more difficult, the behaviour of other people) in the light of what you have found'.

Greenhalgh, 1997

How has Evidence Informed Midwifery Practice?

There are many reasons why midwifery practice should be based on evidence. First and foremost, evidence-based practice is about improving care for women and babies. Sometimes the evidence tells us that the care we have been providing is harmful.

Examples of this include recommending that women eat liver during their pregnancy. This was the norm less than 10 years ago as we believed it would increase women's haemoglobin levels. However later the evidence told us that this was not the case and in fact women should avoid liver because of the potential to overdose on vitamin A. We now know that high dose vitamin A has a potent teratogenic effect and is therefore contra-indicated during pregnancy (Dolk et al, 1999). A further example of a harmful practice is routine episiotomy. The evidence indicated that it is unnecessary to carry out this procedure routinely as episiotomy can cause excess discomfort and delayed perineal healing (Caroli and Belizan, 1999). Similarly, we used to encourage the washing out of babies teats with salt, a practice with the potential to harm babies.

Sometimes the evidence tells us that our practice is ineffectual, such as routine perineal shaving in labour (Vittorio and Lavender, 2007) or giving enemas routinely to women before giving birth (Cuervo, 1999). The most amusing practice which was not based on evidence was removing vases of flowers from postnatal wards at night in the belief that the flowers would eat up all the oxygen.

Equally important is that sometimes the evidence tells us that what we have been doing is right.

As well as improving care, evidence-based practice assists us in ensuring that care is consistent. This is particularly important in busy obstetric units when a woman is likely to receive care from more than one midwife. This does not mean that an individualised approach is not adopted; instead, it means that there is transparency in the care that is given and clear rationales for the care provided. In the current climate of litigation, clear documentation of the evidence drawn upon to guide practice is imperative.

You must also be mindful of the fact that many women clearly want the care they receive to be based on evidence. Furthermore, some women wish to know what that evidence base is. In the small qualitative study by Baker et al (2005), women acknowledged the need for evidence-based care. A midwife who is unable to provide women with the evidence she requests is likely to lose the respect of the woman, which can in turn disrupt the relationship.

How Can you Contribute to Evidence-based Practice?

Each individual has a contribution to make towards evidence-based practice. Importantly this relies on:

- Accessing the best available evidence
- Having clear local and national implementation strategies
- Having defined and appropriate facilitation
- Application of evidence in context
- The involvement of clinicians and consumers.

Several steps illustrate the process of evidence-based practice and how contributions can be made. An individual may contribute to as few or as many parts of the process. Student midwives, are optimally positioned to assimilate information and question practice. Sometimes this questioning can illustrate a lack of understanding of existing evidence or gaps in the available evidence. These gaps can be worked into a formal research question or area of enquiry. These are the main steps to evidence-based practice:

- Converting information needs into focused questions
- Tracking down the best evidence
- Critically appraising the evidence (validity and usefulness)
- Applying results in clinical practice
- Evaluating performance of evidence in clinical application.

If, however, the evidence base is insufficient or not useful further evidence should be recommended.

Implementation

Evidence only becomes useful to practice when implemented. This can be challenging as there are a number of potential barriers. For example, sometimes midwives lack the confidence to challenge the *status quo*. If a practice has continued for some time, and peers are happy with it (for example continuous fetal monitoring), then it is particularly difficult, especially for a junior midwife. However, evidence should be used as a tool to progress; it can in fact give you the strength to challenge.

Another barrier is the fact that as health professionals we do not feel comfortable highlighting the gaps in our knowledge. If we have been providing a particular type of care for some time then we do not want to be told that it has been wrong. For this reason health professionals often 'bury their heads in the sand'.

A further barrier is entrenched views. These entrenched views are born out of traditional beliefs, tribalism, territorialism and selective acceptance of evidence. For example, a midwife may say: '*I know what the evidence says but that study was conducted in London and we are different here in Liverpool.*' Similarly, a midwife may say: '*We have always done it this way and don't see any need to change*'. There are a number of useful steps to implementation (Currie, 2000):

- Identify and engage key individuals, groups, and agencies
- Gain commitment to achieving national standards
- Agree arrangements for implementation
- Set up local implementation teams led by one person who has a clear remit and accountability supported by team members sufficiently senior to commit the organisation to action
- Assess the needs of women and families through community profiling

- Assess existing provision against standards and service models
- Concentrate on the most significant local pressures and gaps, especially those related to workforce, information and leadership
- Agree long-term goals and early measurable deliverables.

Sometimes clinical guidelines are the best way to implement new evidence as these are systematically developed statements designed to support decision making about appropriate healthcare for specific clinical conditions. Rigorously developed, high quality evidence-based guidelines can improve quality of care by improving outcomes, reducing variation in practice, encouraging further research.

The author would like to thank Catherine Ebenezer for her contribution to this chapter.

Activity 6

There is sound evidence that confirms that alternative positions during second stage of labour are favourable for the mother and the baby.

1. Make an observation during your labour ward allocation. How many women adopt alternative positions?

2. Identify reasons why some women adopt them and other women give birth in recumbent position.

NICE guidelines suggests there is no evidence to support continuous fetal monitoring on admission for every woman.

1. Why does this practise still continue?

2. Do you think the evidence detracts from holistic individualised care? Outline the reasons for your opinion.

References

Audit Commission (1997) *First Class Delivery: Improving maternity services in England and Wales*. Audit Commission, London

Baker L, Lavender T, Tincello D (2005) Factors that influence women's decisions about whether to participate in research: an exploratory study. *Birth* **32**(1): 60-66

Besevi V, Lavender T (2006) *Routine perineal shaving on admission in labour.* Cochrane Review, The Cochrane Database of Systematic Reviews Issue 4, 2000

Bewley S, Cockburn J (2002) The unfacts of request Caesarean section. *BJOG* **109**(6): 597-605

Booth A, Dixon-Woods M (2004) *How to do a literature search.* ScHARR, Sheffield. Accessed at: http://www.ccsr.ac.uk/methods/festival2004/programme/Sat/pm/D/Documents/Booth_000.ppt. Accessed on 3 September 2007

Carroli G, Belizan J (1999) *Episiotomy for vaginal birth.* Cochrane Database of Systematic Reviews, Issue 3, 1999

Cuervo LG, Rodríguez MN, Delgado MB (1999) *Enemas during labour.* Cochrane Database of Systematic Reviews 1999, Issue 3, 1999

Currie VL (2000) National Service Frameworks: What are they? *Nursing Standard.* **14**(41): 43-45

Davidoff F, Haynes B, et al (1995) Evidence-Based Medicine. *BMJ* **310**: 1085-1086

Dolk HM, Nau H, Hummlet H, Barlow SM (1999) Dietary vitamin A and teratogenic risk: European Teratology Society discussion paper. *European Journal Obstetrics Gynecology and Reproductive Biology* **83**(1): 31-6

Ebenezer CM (2007) Information: finding the evidence. *RCM Midwives Journal* **10**(9): 434-435

Evans D (2003) Hierarchy of evidence: a framework for ranking evidence evaluating healthcare interventions. *J Clin Nurs* **12**(1): 77-84

Muir Gray JA (1997) *Evidence-based Health Care: How to make health policy and management decisions.* Churchill Livingstone, London

Greenhalgh T (1997) *How to Read a Paper: The basics of evidence-based medicine.* BMJ Publications, London

Kingdon C (2004) Why carry out qualitative research? In: Lavender T et al, eds. *Demystifying Qualitative Research in Pregnancy and Childbirth.* Quay Books, London

Kirkham M (1989) Midwives and information giving during labour. In: Robinson S, Thompson A, eds. *Midwives, Research and Childbirth. Volume 1.* Chapman and Hall, London

Lavender T, Walkinshaw SA (1998) Can midwives reduce postpartum psychological morbidity? A randomized trial. *Birth* **25** (4): 215-9

Lavender T, Hart A, Walkinshaw S, Campbell E, Alfirevic Z (2005) Progress of first stage of labour for multiparous women: an observational study. *BJOG* **112**: 1663-1665

Miller WL, Crabtree (2000) Clinical Research. In: Denzin NK, Lincoln YS, eds. *Handbook of Qualitative Research.* 2nd edition. Sage Publications, London: 607-31

Morgan J (2004) Planning your research. In: Lavender T et al, eds. *Demystifying Qualitative*

Research in Pregnancy and Childbirth. Quay Books, London

Murphey E, Dingwall R, Greatbatch D, Parker S, Watson P (1998) Qualitative methods in health technology assessment: a review of the literature. *Health Technology Assessment* **2**(16): 67

Oakley A (2000) *Experiments in Knowing: Gender and Method in the Social Sciences.* Polity Press, Cambridge

Payton OD (1994) *Research: The Validation of Clinical Practice.* 3rd edn. FA Davis, Philadelphia

Perez-Botella M, Downe S (2006a) Stories as evidence: Why do midwives still use directed pushing? *British Journal of Midwifery* **14**(10): 596–599

Perez-Botella M, Downe S (2006b) Stories as evidence: the premature urge to push. *British Journal of Midwifery* **14**(11): 36 – 642

Popay J, Williams G (1998) Qualitative research and evidence-based healthcare. *Journal of Royal Society of Medicine* **91**(supplement 35): 32-7

Sackett DL, et al (2000) *Evidence-Based Medicine: How to Practice and Teach EBM.* 2nd edition. Churchill Livingstone, Edinburgh

Schardt C, Mayer J (2004) *Introduction to Evidence-based Medicine.* 4th edition. Duke University Medical School, Durham, NC

Snowden C, Elbourne D, Garcia J (2004) Embedding a qualitative approach within a quantitative framework. In: Lavender T et al, eds. *Demystifying Qualitative Research in Pregnancy and Childbirth.* Quay Books, London

Snowden C, Garcia J, Elbourne D (1997) Making sense of randomisation: responses of parents of critically ill babies to random allocation of treatment in a clinical trial. *Soc Sci Med* **45**(9): 1337-55

Waltz C, Bausell RB (1981) *Nursing Research: design, Statistics and Computer Analysis.* Phil. FA Davis Co, Philadelphia

Appendix 1. Useful Sources of Evidence

www..cochrane.org	**The Cochrane Library** This is an electronic publication designed to supply high quality evidence to inform people providing and receiving care, and those responsible for research, teaching, funding and administration at all levels. Cochrane reviews bring you the combined results of the world's best medical research studies, and are recognised as the gold standard in evidence-based health care. Full text articles available for download when accessed via the national NHS e-libraries.
www.rdinfo.org.uk	**RDInfo** RDInfo has become a unique resource dedicated to providing support for UK researchers in the area of health and social care. The unit has gained substantive national recognition and is now responsible for three innovative, interlinked services. Together these cover the fundamental needs of aspiring and experienced researchers by providing health-related research funding opportunities; a telephone signposting service supported by an expert panel (RDDirect); and a directory of health research training.

Continued...

www.york.ac.uk/inst/crd	**Centre for Reviews and Dissemination** This aims to provide research-based information about the effects of interventions used in health and social care. It helps to promote the use of research-based knowledge, by offering: • Rigorous and systematic reviews of research on selected topics • Scoping reviews which map the research literature • Four databases: DARE, NHS EED, the HTA database, and the Ongoing Reviews Database • 'Hitting the Headlines' • Publications: CRD Reports, Effective Health Care, and Effectiveness Matters • A dissemination service • An information and enquiry service
www.rhlibrary.com	**Reproductive Health Library** This assembles the best evidence, categorises treatments by what works and what does not, discusses implications for practice and includes practical resources such as videos and training courses.

Continued...

www.intermid.co.uk	**Intermid** This is the online archive of peer-reviewed midwifery articles published in the *British Journal of Midwifery* and the *African Journal of Midwifery and Women's Health*.
www.internurse.com	**Internurse** This is the online archive of the *British Journal of Nursing* and over 10 other specialist nursing peer-reviewed journals, including the *British Journal of Community Nursing*, and *Practice Nursing*.
www.bjhm.co.uk	***British Journal of Hospital Medicine*** This are the archives of the peer-reviewed *British Journal of Hospital Medicine*. Intermid and Internurse and the *British Journal of Hospital Medicine* are published by MA Healthcare Ltd, the UK's leading independent midwifery and nursing and publisher.
www.aditus.nhs.uk	**Aditus** This is part of the National Library for Health and enables access to bibliographical resources, full-text journal and local resources.

Continued...

www.pubmedcentral.nih.gov	**PubMed Central** This is a free digital archive of biomedical and life sciences journal literature at the US National Institutes of Health (NIH), developed and managed by NIH's National Center for Biotechnology Information (NCBI) in the National Library of Medicine (NLM). It aims to fill the role of a world class library in the digital age. It is not a journal publisher. NLM believes that giving all users free and unrestricted access to the material in PubMed Central is the best way to ensure the durability and utility of the archive as technology changes over time.
www.jr2.ox.ac.uk/Bandolier	**Bandolier** Published in the NHS for the NHS, Bandolier is a newsletter designed to keep purchasers up-to-date with both local and national initiatives and literature on the effectiveness of health care interventions. It is available in full-text and free of charge on the web.

Continued...

www.nrr.nhs.uk	**National Research Register (NRR)** This is a database of ongoing and recently completed research projects funded by, or of interest to, the NHS, produced by Update Software for the Department of Health. The current release contains information on just over 72,000 research projects, as well as entries from the Medical Research Council's Clinical Trials Register, and details on reviews in progress collected by the NHS Centre for Reviews and Dissemination. A key function of the register is to inform researchers, research managers and funders about research that is planned or under way in order to identify gaps and avoid duplication. The complete NRR is now available for free on the web.
www.nice.org.uk	**National Institute for Health and Clinical Excellence (NICE)** NICE is the independent organisation responsible for providing national guidance on the promotion of good health and the prevention and treatment of ill health. NICE produces guidance in three areas of health: 1. Public health 2. Health technologies 3. Clinical practice

CHAPTER 7

Does Litigation Influence Midwifery Practice?

Andrew Symon

In order to address whether litigation affects clinical practice, it is necessary to provide some brief background information on litigation. In this context we mean clinical negligence litigation — the allegation that a practitioner's standard of care fell so far below that which could reasonably be expected, that it led to some kind of harm or damage. There are other forms of litigation in the health service, such as claims dealt with under health and safety or employment law, but we are dealing here with the law of medical negligence. Although the term 'medical' is used, we can substitute the word 'clinical'. Similarly, instead of the word 'negligence' you may see the term 'malpractice' used, although this is usually in US sources.

Claims about a rapid increase in litigation in the UK began to surface in the late 1980s (Ham et al, 1988; MPS, 1989). However, for reasons of commercial confidentiality, the medical defence organisations (MDOs) have not released detailed information on claims data, so the exact picture has been difficult to determine. Nevertheless, local studies have attempted to identify rates for different specialities (e.g. Law et al, 1996), and it was apparent that obstetrics and gynaecology was the specialty most heavily implicated in rising levels of damages; this has recently been confirmed (NHS Litigation Authority [NHSLA], 2006a). Because of the way in which data are reported, it is not possible to say how many midwives have been involved in litigation, and consequently it is difficult to estimate a proportionate response by midwives to the prospect of litigation. My own research into this field involved nearly 1800 midwives and over 200 obstetricians, most of them in Scotland, the remainder being in England. 49% of the obstetricians had been involved in litigation at least once, compared with 4.5% of the midwives. I could not say whether one in twenty or so is an over- or an under-estimate when considering the whole population of midwives in the UK. There are always dangers of bias in any research into such a sensitive subject, of course, but to date there are no other figures detailing midwifery involvement. That imperfect portrayal sets the context for a discussion of whether litigation affects what midwives do.

Defensive Practice

When the fear of litigation is said to influence clinical practice, this is called defensive practice, or sometimes defensive medicine. The latter term gives some indication of where most attention has been focused in recent years concerning this phenomenon — on what doctors do (or do not do) as a result of the fear of being sued. However, there is some evidence that midwives are not immune from this experience. An accepted understanding of defensive medicine is contained in this summary:

> *'The threat of medical malpractice may lead physicians to order medically unnecessary tests and procedures to protect themselves against a future lawsuit.'*
> US Congress, Office of Technology Assessment, 1993

It is evident that this is a description from the USA. However, this should not overshadow the fact that this occurs internationally. The most succinct definition of defensiveness has been given by Black (1990). He characterised defensiveness in terms firstly of risk avoidance, and then of risk reduction. A 'risk avoidance' strategy may include practitioners '... avoiding specialties, procedures, and patients that they perceive carry a high risk of leading to a malpractice claim' (ibid. 36). 'Risk reduction' strategies may include practitioners undertaking 'more investigations and interventions than they would otherwise' (ibid. 36). Very few things in clinical practice are completely standard, and at the time this topic was becoming much talked-about. Clements (1991) noted that 'one man's defensive medicine is another man's risk management'.

Of course, when practitioners are said to be responding to the fear of litigation, this is only one aspect of the process: litigation happens when there are poor clinical outcomes. Most practitioners act and react because they want the clinical outcome to be as good as possible; it may be impossible to identify how much of the decision-making process is affected by medico-legal concerns.

How much evidence is there that defensiveness happens at all? To take the international context to begin with, there have been studies in a number of different countries that report on this. In the USA, Anderson (1999) has reported on the huge costs of defensive medicine — extra tests and investigations do not come cheap. Also in the USA, Studdert et al (2005) report that extra (and often unnecessary) tests are commonplace, and that many doctors avoid certain 'high risk' procedures or patients. Fear of litigation may even affect decisions about resuscitating babies born near the limits of viability (Ballard et al, 2002). In the Netherlands, van Boven et al

(1997) have claimed that there is defensive testing in family practice, and in England Summerton (2000) has reported that GPs have become more likely to carry out investigative tests. In Italy Vimercati et al (2000) have claimed that defensiveness affects all grades of obstetrician in Italy, and there have been concerns expressed in many other countries about the threat of defensive medicine. These include Mexico (Tena Tamayo & Sanchez Gonzalez 2005), France (Guerot 2006) and Switzerland (Junod 2006). It is truly an international phenomenon.

One claim has been that defensiveness has contributed to the rise in caesarean sections, although the evidence for this is debatable. Goyert et al (1989) claim that caesarean rates are not affected by recent medico-legal experience; DeMott and Sandmire (1990) say that such rates reflect an individual's response to the fear of litigation, while Localio et al (1993) state that caesarean rates are positively associated with level of malpractice premiums.

It can be seen that a number of these references are somewhat dated, and this is one of the difficulties in trying to describe accurately what is happening in this area. My own research into this subject took place in the mid-1990s, but with regards to midwifery, there would not appear to be anything more recent to which to point. The following discussion, then, comes with the caveat that the picture may have changed since this research was carried out, but that until someone carries out further studies this is the state of knowledge as it stands.

The whole notion of defensiveness is linked with the possibility of being sued. In order to assess that, you must have some idea of how prevalent litigation is, but here we run into difficulties. It is extremely difficult to identify the incidence of litigation, and for a number of reasons. Historically, claims in England were raised and managed on a regional rather than a national basis, which made collating national data problematic. Different organisations might use different definitions or data standards, and paper records might not be compatible with one another (Vincent et al, 2006). A number of professional defence organisations might be involved, but they rarely published figures because of concerns about commercial sensitivity. In Scotland the claims were all dealt with on a national basis, but the concerns about confidentiality again meant that very few data were published. It must also be borne in mind that the incidence of litigation, set against the total number of adverse outcomes, is low, and that therefore the likelihood of being sued is in fact not great. Negligence law may offer the chance to examine specific instances in great detail, but it cannot provide a systematic analysis of the broader clinical setting to establish why things go wrong (Jones, 2006).

With the advent of the NHS Litigation Authority (NHSLA) in England, national data are now available, but these are reported according to medical specialty, and gynaecological claims are put in together with obstetric ones. For the first eleven years of the new scheme (operated by the Clinical Negligence Scheme for Trusts — CNST), claims concerning obstetrics and gynaecology were the second most common, being 21% of all claims. The most common specialty was surgery, representing 39% of all claims. However, when the claims are presented according to their value (i.e. the potential amounts paid in damages) the picture changes. Obstetrics and gynaecology (which includes midwifery) is by far the most expensive specialty, the main reason being the large amounts of compensation payable in cases involving the long-term care of a child with learning and/or motility disabilities. However, apart from cases reported in the media (e.g. Hall, 2006) and some small-scale studies (Capstick and Edwards, 1990; James, 1991), I found very little precise information about either the incidence or effects of litigation, and it was against this backdrop of partial information that my own research took place in the 1990s.

Asked if they thought litigation was increasing, 90% of the obstetricians and 86% of the midwives in my study agreed. While 76% and 59% respectively thought that practice was becoming defensive, only 43% and 53% of this sample admitted that they had personally changed their practice as a result of the fear of litigation (Symon, 2000a; 2001). There seemed to be an element, then, of practitioners claiming that although they saw their colleagues practising defensively, they were less likely to do this themselves. Asked what constituted defensive practice, the midwives and obstetricians came up with very similar ideas. In fact, the five most commonly cited examples in each group were the same — more Caesareans; earlier intervention; more use of cardiotocography (CTG); more investigations; and more induction of labour. Seventeen percent of the obstetricians admitted that they personally had quicker recourse to caesarean section (a worrying finding in itself), and a small number stated that they intervened more quickly, or requested more investigations, just to be on the safe side. Ten percent said that they documented more, and 5% said that they discussed things more thoroughly with patients, and this raises an interesting issue. Is defensiveness necessarily a bad thing? For the midwives, by far the most common example of a personal change in practice was an increase in the amount of documentation – 42% claimed this. Eight percent said that they now obtained permission for all procedures; 4% referred more quickly to a doctor; 2% adhered more to unit policies; and 1.3% admitted that they used the CTG more often.

Acknowledging the caveats about the timing and location of this study, we can question whether these findings represent a problem for midwifery. We have also to distinguish between those individuals who react in a certain way because they have personally experienced litigation (thankfully a small group in midwifery terms), and those who respond because of a more general fear of litigation. Firstly, to deal with the results from the obstetricians: does it matter if doctors proceed more quickly to caesarean section? Yes, it does, because some of these will be unnecessary caesareans, and that is in no one's interests. However, it is hard to see that doctors writing more in the case notes, or discussing things in more detail with pregnant women, are a bad thing. Likewise, for midwives to be documenting more does not seem to represent a crisis (although more is not necessarily better), and if more midwives are obtaining permission for the procedures they carry out, it is hard to portray that as a problem. Although in general terms, then, it is difficult to point to a crisis in clinical practice for maternity care; it is worth examining how some individuals have reacted. The intention here is to help identify potential problem areas, so that individuals can work out how best to respond in a similar situation.

Case Studies

As previously reported (Symon, 2000b), one midwifery manager told me:

'We had one consultant who induced everybody, everybody on the dot, at forty weeks ... Something in the past, you know, he had a bad experience.'

Symon, 2000b

When there is a catastrophic clinical outcome, it is perfectly natural to react in a way that is intended to minimise the risk of a recurrence. To an extent, this kind of reaction has been mitigated by the growth in unit protocols, which are discussed later on in this chapter. It is sad, however, to note the detrimental effect such a reaction would have on others: while difficult to quantify, it can be seen that for every baby saved by such a response, there would be many other instances where unnecessary interventions would ensue. It is easy to see how routine inductions will often become failed inductions: the 'cascade of intervention' has been well documented (Tracy and Tracy, 2003). Again, at interview (Symon 2000b) one obstetrician noted:

'In the past where one might have reviewed a situation, had another look, now I think we would probably do a Caesar. But ... (obstetricians) are not doing a Caesar for litigation, they're doing a Caesar to get the baby out, but I think the threat of litigation is always there at the back of one's mind.'

Symon, 2000b

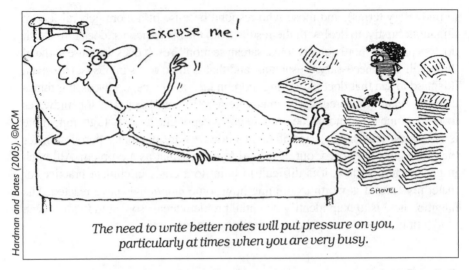

Hardman and Bates (2005). ©RCM

The need to write better notes will put pressure on you, particularly at times when you are very busy.

This brings us to the matter of decision-making. In a clinical situation, particularly one that is moving quickly, decisions may have to be made rapidly. Experience counts, as do the particular clinical findings and the local circumstances. It is very difficult to verify just how much of the decision is affected by the fear that, somewhere down the line, a lawyer is going to be poring over the case notes. However, as this obstetrician has noted, it is there somewhere in the thinking. Practitioners have to be aware of how and why they arrive at a certain decision in order to know whether it is justified.

As for midwives writing more in the case notes, this ought to be a positive thing, and may be something that comes with experience. It can be difficult to know just how much detail is required when completing case notes: what is essential, and what is not? One midwife who had been involved in litigation noted (Symon, 2001):

> *'I just think I've increased the amount of documentation I do — but not since the court case. This has been my progression, sort of growing up as a midwife.'*
>
> Symon, 2001

In her case she was sure that her reasons for writing more were not due to the experience of being involved in a legal claim. Another midwife admitted that (Symon, 2001):

> *'There are times when I think we're writing far more and not giving as much physical support. When you go in to see somebody, instead of rubbing her back you're scribbling in the notes.'*
>
> Symon, 2001

In this case, the desire to produce apparently good-looking case notes superseded the professional impulse to provide good care. That this was not that unusual an example was confirmed by a representative from a consumer organisation, who told me (Symon, 2000b):

> *'You get these beautifully documented notes where (the midwives) write everything down beautifully in longhand, and essentially what they're doing is writing down that the baby died, but they're not actually doing anything about it.'*

Symon, 2000b

Clearly the cart is before the horse in a situation like this: the care should always come first. There is a balance to be struck, but it is important to get this balance right. A midwifery lecturer confirmed to me that students sometimes find this difficult (Symon, 2000b):

> *'I did a seminar (with student midwives) and said "What is the reason for record keeping?" And the response was "Fear of litigation". Their thoughts were "We only keep records because we might be called to account." Litigation should be at the bottom of the list; something to remember, but not the prime reason.'*

Symon, 2000b

Another midwife pointed out to me the dangers of giving clinical care that is procedure-focused rather than woman-focused. She noted (Symon, 2000b):

> *'(Litigation) probably means you're practising more defensively, where before you could treat people as individuals and adapt your practice to suit the individual ... Now there maybe is a tendency to control from a policy document.'*

Symon, 2000b

This brings us onto the question of how the health service has tried to deal with the problem of litigation.

Clinical Governance and Risk Management

Clinical governance can be seen as the strategic umbrella which covers risk management together with fitness for practise and clinical effectiveness. Introduced in 1997, many have noted that most aspects of clinical governance are not actually new; they have simply been re-branded. What was new was that the new governance framework placed a statutory duty on the health service to comply with its requirements (Harrison et al 2003).

'Fitness for practise' covers such aspects as life-long learning, continuing professional development, professional revalidation and managing poor performance. 'Clinical effectiveness' incorporates critical appraisal, evidence-based practice, standards and guidelines, audit and research, outcome indicators and integrated care pathways. These two areas are dealt with briefly at the end of this section. However, it is risk management which is perhaps best known in a medico-legal context, and with which we are most concerned here. Its medico-legal origins are noted by Walshe and Sheldon (1998), who state:

'It has been largely the financial pressure from legal actions for clinical negligence which has driven the NHS to take risk and risk management seriously.'

Walshe and Sheldon, 1998

Whatever the original impetus towards risk management, it now covers financial and health and safety concerns, as well as clinical issues.

While many of the concepts of risk management have been part of sound clinical practice for many years, its formal introduction into clinical care has not been without criticism. There are those, for instance, who see it as a potential control tool for managers and clinicians (Edwards and Murphy-Lawless, 2006). We should be careful about assuming that we can actually manage risk; we are certainly not always good at predicting it. Even the best risk-prediction schemes fail to identify every problem. However, risk management is the attempt to control difficult clinical situations. From a fairly straightforward concept of identifying what goes wrong and trying to find out how to address this problem, it has developed into a more complex system covering organisational culture, learning from mistakes, training, guideline development, and claims and complaints management. This is in part due to the recognition that although individual practitioners make mistakes, the system in which they work can be seen to pre-dispose them to making such mistakes.

Reason (2001) claims that practitioners are 'the inheritors rather than the instigators of an accident sequence'; in other words they make mistakes partly because the conditions are right for them to do so. What this means in terms of developing risk management is that in addition to ensuring that practitioners are well trained and kept up-to-date in their skills, the organisational conditions that predispose towards errors are also addressed. These conditions might include chronic staffing shortages; poor workload management; a poor skill mix in critical areas like labour ward, resulting in inexperienced staff receiving inadequate supervision. In addition, the culture of a unit can contribute to poor outcomes if effective communication is discouraged, perhaps because of rigid hierarchical structures, or if there is a reluctance to admit to certain problems, whether individual or organisational.

There are issues, too, to do with blaming. Accountability is a central feature of professionalism, but we can ask how much blame is necessary in order for practitioners to be accountable. Some would like to see a 'blame-free' approach as a means of encouraging practitioners to be completely open about the mistakes they make, but it is acknowledged that this may deny part of the core of accountability (McNeill and Walton, 2002). Midwives have admitted to failing to admit to their own errors, and to covering up for their colleagues on occasion (Symon et al, 2006). While understandable, it can be questioned where this leaves notions of professional accountability.

Essentially, risk management aims to identify risk; assess it; and take action to reduce it. To this end, national Risk Management Standards have been developed for different clinical areas, including maternity care. These are considered in the next section.

'Clinical Effectiveness' is one of the key elements in the model of clinical governance. It has been an important platform for the promotion of up-to-date clinical practices. It was used in relation to medical practice initially but has a much broader application to other professions in health care. It requires the implementation of evidence-based practice to promote clinically effective and cost effective care. Again, this may be portrayed in terms of using standards and protocols. Essentially it is about using the best available evidence to make decisions about clinical practice and then to change that practice in line with the evidence. The final stage in this process is to determine whether or not the change has been effective (Weston et al, 2001).

'Fitness for Practise' also sits under the Clinical Governance umbrella, and 'life-long learning' is one of its aims. For example, in Scotland the *Learning Together* document (Scottish Executive, 1999) states that learning is vital in order to deliver high quality, responsive care, and delivering high quality care requires that high standards are achieved and maintained through continuous improvement. The changes necessary to meet these requirements need staff 'with flexible skills and the support to maximise their potential' (Scottish Executive, 1999).

Post-Registration Education and Practice (PREP) addresses issues of continuing professional development, professional regulation and lifelong learning. Other professions have equivalent processes for continuing professional development and many are currently under review. It is worth noting that, although the fundamentals of midwifery do not change, the context may do, and some of what is learnt in a pre-registration programme may become obsolete. Only by continuing to learn throughout our professional lives can we hope to maintain the necessary standards of professional practice (NMC, 2002). Partly because of the transitory nature of some of what is learnt, 'Fitness for Practise' also concerns revalidation; this has resulted from public and professional concerns about maintaining up-to-date knowledge, attitudes and skills. How poor performance is managed is more difficult, sometimes because we are not always clear about the standards against which we are measuring performance. It is reasonably easy to recognise poor performance in specific activities, such as the prescription and administration of medicines where there are very clear criteria on performance, but more difficult to do so, for example, in the case of woman whose labour is being augmented, and whose CTG trace is questionable. In such a scenario there may be doubt as to exactly when it is correct to intervene.

CNST / CNORIS / Welsh Risk Pool

Health care is a devolved matter in political terms: since the re-convening of the Scottish parliament in 1999, and the inauguration of the Welsh Assembly in the same year, health care matters in Scotland and Wales have been managed by those institutions. In Northern Ireland, the relevant department under the devolved assembly there is the Department of Health, Social Services and Public Safety. This means that a description of what happens in England may not hold true for the other countries within the UK, although the broad thrust of health policy is similar. In England the NHS Litigation Authority (NHSLA) was set up as a Special Health Authority responsible for handling both clinical and non-clinical negligence cases on behalf of the NHS in England. It notes:

> *'Clinical claims arising out of incidents occurring after 1 April 1995 are handled under the 'Clinical Negligence Scheme for Trusts' (CNST), a voluntary risk-pooling scheme for NHS trusts, Foundation trusts and PCTs [Primary Care Trusts]. Claims relating to incidents from before April 1995 are handled under the "Existing Liabilities Scheme'"(ELS), now funded centrally by the Department of Health.'*

NHSLA 2006a

Although initially membership of CNST was voluntary, by 31st March 2005 all Foundation Trusts, NHS Trusts and PCTs were members.

In Scotland the equivalent of CNST is the Clinical Negligence and Other Risks Indemnity Scheme (CNORIS), which produced risk management standards for Scotland; these were recently merged with the Clinical Governance Standards developed by NHS Quality Improvement Scotland (NHS QIS). Membership of CNORIS has been mandatory for all health bodies since its inception in 2000; it deals with all claims relating to the NHS in Scotland.

In Wales, the Welsh Risk Pool is the equivalent. It is a mutual organisation that pools resources from its member organisations in order to cover the costs of negligence actions. In Northern Ireland, the Department of Health, Social Services and public Safety handles such matters.

Individual hospitals will be expected to adhere to the standards produced by these bodies in order to reduce their insurance premiums, the insurance being against future litigation. As part of this overall strategy, there would usually be a documented policy on risk, and written policies or guidelines for staff to follow in relation to particular risks, such as accidents, needle stick injuries and clinical errors. Policies and protocols are discussed further in the next section.

In order to demonstrate that individual hospitals have taken on board the need to reduce the likelihood of poor outcomes, and to mitigate the effects of outcomes that are poor, the CNST Standards (NHSLA, 2006b) require that hospitals address a number of areas under the following headings:

1: Organisation
2: Learning from Experience
3: Communication
4: Clinical Care
5: Induction, Training and Competence
6: Health Records
7: Implementation of Clinical Risk Management
8: Staffing Levels

These would encompass such things as ensuring that the policy relating to maternity clinical risk management specifies who is responsible for the woman's care at all times, and that there are referenced, evidence-based multidisciplinary policies for the management of all key procedures or situations during labour. A system for reporting and analysing clinical incidents should also be in place. The intention is to manage and control some of the vagaries of clinical practice, particularly in the acute setting. One of the ways in which it attempts to do this is now considered.

Policies and Protocols

We have seen that policies and protocols are one way in which institutions attempt to minimise the risk of poor outcomes. On the one hand, having a uniform policy in a unit presents the possibility of a certain equity of service. Women are treated equally, which circumvents the dangers that were inherent in the past when there were as many different régimes for induction of labour as there were consultant obstetricians in that unit — a recipe for mistakes, as junior staff misapplied instructions. On the other hand, the notion that 'one-size-fits-all' hardly sits comfortably with the idea of individualised care. There are dangers in trying to make women fit the protocol: even when evidence-based (as all protocols should be), the evidence base on which they rest will be partial. No research study covers every situation, but will make recommendations based on the results it was able to obtain.

To try and get around this, there are different levels of recommendation. The language used can be very instructive. For instance, NICE (2006) states its guideline on postnatal care has been developed with the following aims:

'To advise on appropriate objectives, purpose, content and timing of postnatal contacts and care for the woman and her baby;

'To advise on best practices and competencies for assessment of postnatal health and management of postnatal problems in the woman and/or her infant;

'To advise on information, education and support required during the postnatal period;

'To advise on planning of postnatal care;

'To consider good practice in communication between health care providers and women, their partners and other family members.'

NICE, 2006

Note the lack of specific instruction: the guideline advises and gets practitioners to consider. Contrast this with the RCOG's (2001) *'Indications for the use of continuous electronic fetal monitoring'* (EFM): 'Continuous EFM should be used where oxytocin is being used for induction or augmentation of labour.'

The difference in language is explained by the different levels of evidence on which the various guidelines are based: well-designed controlled studies, ideally with randomisation, are said to justify a more instructive term such as 'should'.

There are inherent difficulties here: what if a practitioner decides that he/she does not want to follow the protocol? What if the woman herself indicates that she does not want it to be followed? In the latter case there is little doubt in a legal sense: as long as the woman is mentally competent, she can refuse any form of treatment or intervention, even if that is thought likely to lead to her death or that of her unborn baby. Such extreme cases are rare, but the principle is clear: the woman has the right to determine what happens to her body. What, then, of the practitioner who decides not to follow a protocol? In a legal sense it has been noted that as no two legal claims will be exactly the same, and as guidance will change over time there can be no hard and fast rules as to whether not following guidance is acceptable (Airedale NHS Trust *v* Bland 1993). Practitioners who face allegations of negligence will be judged by what is known as the 'Bolam test' (or 'Hunter *v* Hanley test' in Scotland). This states that a practitioner's actions in England, Wales and Northern Ireland are safe as long as they are in accordance with a reasonable body of opinion. In Scotland the action is safe unless it is shown that no practitioner of ordinary skill would have acted in the way alleged. In other words, protocols or guidelines do not replace this need to establish, usually by expert opinion, that an action or omission was acceptable or not. Lee (2000) notes that: 'It is not enough for the patient's barrister to simply wave some guidelines in front of the court and say "*I rest my case, your honour*". The guidelines have to be part of accepted practice.'

What should you do, then, in relation to unit protocols? The good news is that most of the ones developed for midwifery practice (e.g. RCM, 2005) have a sound evidence base and can be trusted, so you should feel confident about following them. Most guideline development groups now are concerned to ensure that they reflect user opinion where once this was either completely absent or felt by some to be tokenism (Symon, 2001). Remember always that care should be individualised and that there may be a reason why the protocol does not fit a particular woman. With greater experience and confidence comes the ability to make such judgement calls.

Complaints

The difficulties with identifying precise figures for litigation have been noted above. Complaints may be seen as another sub-set of expressions of dissatisfaction, but their relationship with legal claims is impossible to verify. Certainly a complaint is less serious than a legal claim in terms of involvement and likely consequences, but that does not mean that incidents that lead to complaints are necessarily less serious than those incidents which form the basis of a legal claim. Both avenues are open to disgruntled service users, and it is not known why some people go down one route, and some the other.

While the overall incidence of complaints has been much easier to identify than the incidence of litigation, the same problems about aggregated data exist, and it is not possible to identify exactly how many complaints relate to midwives. After several years of claims about rising complaints levels (Warden, 1996; Dunne, 1999; Remmers, 2002), there would appear to have been a slight fall in numbers (Symon, 2006). However, there are too many examples of women suffering because of poor clinical care and subsequent ineffectual communication (Robinson, 2005) for midwives to be complacent. For the year up to March 2004 there were approximately 3,000 complaints concerning maternity care (Symon, 2006); it is not known how many related specifically to midwives. I believe most midwives pride themselves on being good communicators, but poor communication is a common feature in many complaints (HSO, 2003).

Advice for patients who want to make a complaint against the NHS is provided by the Ombudsman (PHSO, 2006). A complaint can be made by anyone affected or likely to be affected by a practitioner's actions or decisions, and should normally be made within six months. Many complaints concern poor communication, either with the woman and her family, or between practitioners; poor staffing levels are also a common feature, as is the attitude shown by staff (Sidgewick, 2006). Many of those who complain are said to want an explanation and perhaps an apology; sometimes they may want reassurance that similar mistakes or outcomes will be avoided in the future.

There will be a designated Complaints Officer where you work, and the complaints procedure aims to deal with matters locally if possible. However, any member of staff may be contacted in the first instance; this may be when someone turns up where you work, or telephones in. If this happens, you should politely note down the details, and say that you will contact the unit's Complaints Officer. If 'Local Resolution' does not satisfy the person complaining, the complaint can be made formally to the organisation. If they are still not satisfied, they can request an independent review by the Ombudsman, although comparatively few are taken this far. If you have been personally involved in an incident about which a complaint is made, you may be required to write a statement. Such statements are used to investigate the matter in detail, and provide the Complaints Officer with the information required to address the issue. An example of a statement writing template is given by the Royal College of Midwives (RCM 1997) — see Appendix 1 at the end of this chapter.

The procedures for dealing with complaints is generally to be open and sympathetic. It is perhaps surprising, certainly depressing, to note that the complaints process can at times make people more, not less, angry (PHSO, 2005).

From the information available, it would appear that litigation probably does influence midwifery practice, but for a number of reasons this is difficult to quantify. While maternity care is one of the most common areas for negligence claims (and it is certainly the most expensive specialty in terms of compensation payouts), midwives have been much less involved in litigation than obstetricians. There is little information detailing actual figures about midwifery involvement in litigation, so it is difficult to know what a proportionate response would be in any case. In addition, not all the claimed consequences of litigation are necessarily negative — if practitioners are discussing more with those under their care and writing better notes, it can be argued that the standard of care has been improved. Of course, it is possible to see adverse outcomes too: over-investigating and intervening too quickly are undesirable consequences of this phenomenon, since both reduce choice and may in fact lead to increased morbidity.

Litigation and complaints are features of accountability — a crucial aspect of professionalism — and it can be argued that they offer an opportunity for the profession to identify and address problems in clinical practice. The way the health service has approached this is in the guise of healthcare governance, and specifically risk management. Getting the balance right between using evidence-based guidelines and providing sensitive individualised care may be tricky at times, but as students remember that you should have the support of clinical mentors and academic lecturers. There is help and guidance available if you do happen to be involved in an untoward incident and are asked to write a statement.

Activity 7

1. Explore the complaints procedures in your unit. Have you encountered any experiences where midwives have been asked to write a statement in response to a complaint made by a user of the service?

2. What are your views when an individual professional is targeted for statement writing when a whole team has been responsible for delivery of care?

3. Do you think increased litigation promotes defensive practice? Support your answers with examples.

References

Anderson RE (1999) Billions for defense: the pervasive nature of defensive medicine. *Archives of Internal Medicine* **159**(20): 2399–402

Ballard DW, Li Y, Evans J et al (2002) Fear of litigation may increase resuscitation of infants born near the limits of viability. *J Pediatrics* **140**(6): 713–18

Black N (1990) Medical Litigation and the quality of care. *Lancet* **335**(8680): 35-7

Capstick JB, Edwards PJ (1990) Trends in obstetric malpractice claims. *Lancet* **336**(8720): 931–2

Clements R (1991) Litigation in obstetrics and gynaecology. *British Journal of Obstetrics and Gynaecology* **98:** 423–6

DeMott RK, Sandmire HF (1990) The Green Bay cesarean section study I. The physical factor as a determinant of Caesarean birth rates. *American Journal of Obstetrics and Gynecology* **162**(6): 1593–602

Dunne R (1999) GMC to clear jam of complaints. *Hospital Doctor* **12/8/99:** 3

Edwards N, Murphy-Lawless J (2006) The Instability of Risk: Women's Perspectives on Risk and Safety in Birth. In: Symon A ed. *Risk and Choice in Maternity Care*. Elsevier, Edinburgh

Goyert G, Bottoms S, Treadwell M et al (1989) The physician factor in cesarean birth rates. *New England Journal of Medicine* **320**(11): 706–9

Guerot C (2006) Medical liability: moving forward. *Presse Medicale* **35**(6 Pt 2): 1031–4

Hall S (2006) Millions for boy, eight, brain-damaged at birth. *Guardian* **11th May:**

Ham C, Dingwall R, Fenn P (1988) *Medical Negligence: Compensation and Accountability*. King's Fund Institute, London

Hrdman L, Bates C (2005) *Litigation: A Risk Management Guide for Midwives*. 2nd edn. RCM Trust, London

Harrison S, Pollock C, Symons S (2003) *Getting to grips with Clinical Governance*. TFM Publishing, Harley

HSO [Health Service Ombudsman for England] (2003) *Annual Report 2002-3*. HMSO, London

James C (1991) Risk Management in obstetrics and gynaecology. *Journal of the Medical Defence Union* **7:** 36–8

Jones M (2006) Patient safety and the law. In: Walshe K, Broaden R eds. *Patient Safety: research into practice*. OUP, Maidenhead

Junod AF (2006) Les pratiques medicales defensives aux Etats-Unis. A quand la Suisse? *Revue Medicale Suisse* **2**(54): 552

Law D, Lewington T, Fletcher R et al (1996) Allegations of Medical Negligence against Hospitals in the West Midlands Region. *Journal of the Medical Defence Union* **12**(3): 67–9

Lee R (2000) A guide to guidelines. *Journal of the Medical Defence Union* **16**(1): 23–4

Localio A, Lawthers A, Bengtson J et al (1993) Relationship between malpractice claims and cesarean delivery. *Journal of the American Medical Association* **269**(3): 366–73

McNeill PM, Walton M (2002) Medical harm and the consequences of error for doctors. *Medical Journal of Australia* **176**(5): 222–5

MPS (1989) *Annual Report*. Medical Protection Society, London

NHSLA [NHS Litigation Authority] (2006a) Factsheet 3: information on claims. NHSLA, London

NHSLA (2006b) Clinical Negligence Scheme for Trusts- Maternity Clinical Risk Management Standards. www.nhsla.com/NR/rdonlyres/002DB3DE-F1A1-4153-AFE1-B59A3D743239/0/CNSTMaternityStandardsApril2006final.pdf

NICE [National Institute for health and Clinical Excellence] (2006) Postnatal care: Routine postnatal pare of women and their babies. http://www.nice.org.uk/page.aspx?o=cg37full guideline. (accessed 28/09/06)

NMC [Nursing & Midwifery Council] (2002) PREP handbook. NMC, London

PHSO [Parliamentary and Health Service Ombudsman for England] (2005) *A Guide to Making a Complaint Against the NHS, a Government Department or Agency.* PHSO, London

PHSO (2006) A guide to making a complaint against the NHS, a government department or agency. www.ombudsman.org.uk/make_a_complaint/parliamentary/guide_to_make_a_complaint.html

RCM [Royal College of Midwives] (1997) Statement writing: what is required in a statement. RCM, London www.rcm.org.uk/info/docs/Statement%20writing.doc

RCM (2005) Evidence based Guidelines for Midwifery-led care in labour. RCM, London

RCOG [Royal College of Obstetricians and Gynaecologists] (2001) The Use of Electronic Fetal Monitoring The use and interpretation of cardiotocography in intrapartum fetal surveillance. Evidence-based Clinical Guideline Number 8. RCOG, London

Reason J (2001) Understanding adverse events: the human factor. In: Vincent C ed. *Clinical risk management: enhancing patient safety* 2nd edn. BMJ Books, London

Remmers A (2002) Who's complaining now? *MIDIRS Midwifery Digest* **12**(3): 412–4

Robinson J (2005) Complaints and forgiveness: the healing process. *British Journal of Midwifery* **13**(4): 243

Scottish Executive (1999) *Learning Together.* Scottish Executive Health Department, Edinburgh

Sidgewick C (2006) Everybody's business: managing midwifery complaints. *British Journal of Midwifery* **14**(2): 70–1

Studdert DM, Mello MM, Sage WM et al (2005) Defensive medicine among high-risk specialist physicians in a volatile malpractice environment. *JAMA* **293**(21): 2609–17

Summerton N (2000) Trends in negative defensive medicine within general practice. *British Journal of General Practice* **50**(456): 565–6

Symon A (2000a) Litigation and defensive clinical practice: quantifying the problem. *Midwifery* **16**(1): 8–14

Symon A (2000b) Litigation and changes in professional behaviour: a qualitative appraisal. *Midwifery* **16**(1): 15–21

Symon A (2001) *Obstetric Litigation from A-Z.* Quay Books, Salisbury

Symon A (2006) Are we facing a complaints and litigation crisis in the health service? *British Journal of Midwifery* **14**(3): 164–5

Symon A, Murphy-Black T, McStea B (2006) An exploratory mixed-methods study of

Scottish midwives' understandings and perceptions of clinical near misses in maternity care. *Midwifery* **22**(2): 125–36

Tena Tamayo C, Sanchez Gonzalez JM. (2005) Assertive medicine: a proposal against defensive medicine. *Ginecologia y Obstetricia de Mexico* **73**(10): 553–9

Tracy SK, Tracy MB (2003) Costing the cascade: estimating the cost of increased obstetric intervention in childbirth using population data. *BJOG* **110**(8): 717–24

van Boven K, Dijksterhuis P, Lamberts H (1997) Defensive testing in Dutch family practice. Is the grass greener on the other side of the ocean? *Journal of Family Practice* **44**(5): 468–72

Vimercati A, Greco P, Loizzi V et al (2000) "Defensive medicine" in the choice of cesarean section. *Acta Bio-Medica de l Ateneo Parmense* **71**(Suppl. 1): 717–21

Vincent C, Walshe K, Davy C et al (2006) Learning from litigation. In: Walshe K, Broaden R eds. *Patient Safety: research into practice*. OUP, Maidenhead

Walshe K, Sheldon T (1998) Dealing with clinical risk: implications of the rise of evidence-based health care. *Public Money and Management* **18**(4): 15–20

Warden J (1996) NHS repeats its mistakes. *British Medical Journal* **312**(7041): 1247

Weston A, Chambers R, Boath E (2001) *Clinical Effectiveness and Clinical Governance for Midwives*. Radcliffe Medical Press, Abingdon

Legal cases

Airedale NHS Trust *v* Bland (1993) 1 All ER 821

Bolam *v* Friern HMC 1957 2 All ER 118

Hunter *v* Hanley 1955 SC 200

Appendix 1. Statement Writing Template (RCM, 1997)

HOW TO WRITE A STATEMENT

A statement should include the following information:

- Full name, qualifications (with dates), status, length of employment at the time of the incident and also at present if this is now different
- Relevant period of duty
- Relate any exceptional points (i.e. ward in process of redecoration, etc)
- A factual narrative of your role in woman's care, making it clear which parts are constructed from memory, the client's records or from your recollection of standard practice at the time
- No statement should be written entirely from memory. Reference should always be made to the client's notes
- Identify other staff involved in the client's care if possible, especially if the signatures are illegible
- Your comments on any allegations concerning your involvement that may have already been made on behalf of the woman
- Each page should have your signature and date of signing. Sign the last page at the end of the text and not at the bottom of the page. Any alterations should also be signed and dated
- You cannot refuse to make a statement but you can insist on time to seek professional advice and assistance in writing your statement

DO REMEMBER

- Be completely honest and state if you cannot remember something
- Avoid ambiguity
- Avoid opinion; state facts only
- Avoid abbreviations
- Explain why you made the decisions you did or took a particular form of action
- Retain a copy for yourself

DO NOT

- Simply repeat what is written in the records; you must expand on what is documented there
- Include opinions or speculations on what other people were doing — include factual information only
- Attempt to write a statement without access to the records and copy of the CTG tracing if applicable
- Write a statement in a hurry; always seek advice.

CHAPTER 8

Changing Social and Political Constructs: Impact on the Role of the Midwife

Carol Bates

British society underwent tremendous change throughout the twentieth century as the western world moved rapidly towards a technological age. This impacted upon all aspects of life in the UK, including the nature of maternity care. This profoundly affected women's experience of childbearing and the role and activities of the midwife.

Two World Wars also changed the nature of society in Britain and as society changed so social mores changed. Contraception, especially oral contraception gave women (and men) greater sexual freedom and by the 1970s legislation had legalised homosexuality (1967) and made abortion (1967) and divorce (1969) more freely available.

Family structures changed significantly as divorce and consequently lone parent rates increased, the popularity of marriage declined as more couples chose to live together and single motherhood became the norm. Legislation enabled gay couples to enter civil partnerships and adopt children. Whilst the overall birth rate declined (Oakley, 1992), teenage pregnancy rates significantly increased in the western world with the UK having the highest rate in Europe (Chambers et al, 2001; Dennison, 2004).

The century saw increasing conflict and war in various parts of the world. Millions of people became homeless and poverty stricken, which resulted in a migration of peoples seeking sanctuary and political asylum in the West. The European Community also continued to expand and consequently the UK became a more complex society in relation to class, culture, race and ethnicity.

Overall, childbirth became safer and as it moved from the private to the public sphere, society's attitudes and women's views on childbirth changed significantly. For example, at the turn of the 20th century women were campaigning for the right to a hospital birth, whilst at the turn of the 21st century women are campaigning for the right to a home birth.

Factors such as family planning, the Abortion Act, antenatal screening, the development of fetal medicine and the increasingly sophisticated nature of the reproductive technologies, for example, In Vitro Fertilisation (IVF) techniques, the human genome project and stem cell research have further changed both women and men's attitudes towards pregnancy and childbirth and consequently expectations have also changed.

Pregnancy and birth became a marketable commodity and there is now a plethora of publications about pregnancy, birth and parenting along with numerous internet websites. Many couples expect pregnancy and birth to be a shared experience that is both psychologically and emotionally fulfilling.

But this is not the case for all women. The rate of postnatal depression had remained constant at around 10% of women for many years but a meta-analysis of the postnatal depression rate (O'Hara and Swain, 1996) showed that by the 1990s the rate had increased to 13% of women, and according to NICE guideline 45: antenatal and postnatal mental health (NICE, 2007) this has further increased to include between 15% and 20% of women in the first 12 months following the birth of their child.

The role of the midwife continually changed throughout the century and whilst the overall position of women in society improved, the same cannot be said for midwives' as a group. Our status did not improve because the sophisticated nature of technology relating to all aspects of fertility ensured that obstetrics remained the dominant discourse. The challenge for midwives in the twenty first century is to open up options and choices for women and to do that effectively perhaps we need to learn lessons from the past.

Changing Context of Midwifery Practice

The last hundred years has seen profound changes in the context of midwifery practice. Change became inevitable as the government addressed public health issues and scientific knowledge progressed. Maternity care expanded as doctors became increasingly involved in the provision of care and place of birth was gradually transferred from home to hospital.

The passing of the first Midwives Act (1902) in Scotland (1915) introduced statutory control of midwifery practice and defined the sphere of midwifery practice to normal pregnancy, labour and birth although this included breech and twin births. Maternal and infant mortality rates were very high and the drive for midwifery registration was seen as an important component of the drive to improve maternal and child health. By 1936 the transition from independent midwifery practice to state salaried employment was complete.

The Act also provided for state registration and mandatory training of midwives. It established the setting up of the Central Midwives Board (CMB) and the regulations for the training and supervision of midwifery practice.

The introduction of the National Health Service (NHS) in 1948 had a profound impact on midwives working patterns that were to continue throughout the 20th and into the 21st century. There were now two distinct groups of midwives. The domiciliary or district midwife employed by the local authority and the hospital midwife employed by the NHS.

Women now had the opportunity for a hospital confinement and ultimately this resulted in fragmentation of care and fundamentally affected the role of the domiciliary midwife once the majority of women gave birth in hospital.

During the 1950s, the homebirth rate dropped significantly and this trend continued at a pace following publication of the Cranbrook Committee Report (HMSO, 1959) which recommended a 70 % hospital confinement rate. The Peel Report (DHSS, 1970) went a step further and recommended a 100% hospital confinement in the interests of safety of mother and baby. This further fragmented midwifery care and enabled the medicalisation of childbirth to begin in earnest. The care women received began to be based upon the obstetric rationale that childbirth could only be considered normal in retrospect and women were placed into high and low risk categories.

The trend from community-based care to hospital based consultant led care had an enormous impact on the work of midwives. Home Births almost disappeared and midwifery skills became devalued in favour of an interventionist approach to care. Some midwives embraced the changes because it meant shorter working hours with less responsibility but others remained dissatisfied and a small number took up independent practice.

A group of student midwives expressed their dissatisfaction by setting up the Radical Midwives Association in 1976 to actively campaign for less intervention and a return of traditional midwifery skills but the interventionist approach continued and following publication of the Short Report on perinatal and neonatal mortality (HMSO, 1980) the routine application of technology intensified throughout the 1980s.

The use of ultrasound became integrated into antenatal care and antenatal screening became increasingly sophisticated. From hereon obstetricians had two patients, mother and fetus and the drive to reduce perinatal mortality rates underpinned maternity care.

Despite childbirth becoming safer, women became increasingly dissatisfied with the routine, depersonalized maternity care they received and consumer groups such as the National Childbirth Trust and the Association for Improvements in Maternity Services campaigned relentlessly on behalf of childbearing women. This culminated in a House of Commons Select Committee chaired by Nicholas Winterton. For the first time midwives were among those groups asked to give evidence to the Select Committee. The report of this committee (House of Commons, 1992) highlighted the importance of the social context of childbearing and the impact of health inequalities. The report expressed the view that the outcome of pregnancy for both mother and baby was largely dependent on the woman's social environment and it questioned the indiscriminate use of technology that had become the norm.

On the strength of this report, the government convened another committee chaired by Baroness Cumberlege. The report of this committee *Changing Childbirth* (DH, 1993), recommended women had choice and greater control of the childbearing process. This included choice in relation to place of birth and a choice of lead professional for their maternity care. A woman could choose midwife, GP or consultant-led care. The other three countries of the UK also reviewed their provision of maternity care and published reports that supported giving women greater choice and control of the care they received (Welsh Office, 1991; Scottish Office, 1993; DHSS Northern Ireland, 1994). These four reports brought a wind of change to the maternity services throughout the UK. Midwives sought opportunities to rethink models of midwifery care in an effort to provide a degree of continuity of care for women within a fragmented service and to restore a degree of autonomy to midwifery practice. Midwives began to adopt different ways of working in a variety of clinical settings; consultant led units; midwife led units and birth centres and the home birth rate began to rise.

Social Profile of Student Midwives in the 21st Century

The social profile of student midwives has changed considerably. Until the passing of the Midwives Act (1902) the concept of the student midwife did not exist. Before the 1902 midwifery skills were acquired through experience and an informal apprenticeship. Often skills were passed on from mother to daughter. Although there were many midwives who did not have any formal training, some midwives offered apprenticeships (for payment) which could last as long as seven years (Oakley, 1976).

At the turn of the 20th century the pupil midwife (the term student midwife was not used until the 1970s) was likely to be married but once trained nurses began to enter midwifery training in 1929, the majority of pupil midwives were young, single women without children. This trend continued until the increased availability of direct entry or pre registration midwifery education programmes began to attract older women with children in the late 1980s.

A Royal College of Midwives (RCM) survey of student midwives for the RCM Student Midwives Hardship Campaign confirms this change (RCM 2004). The survey demonstrated the much broader age range of present day student midwives and more than half of student midwives have children.

Midwifery remains a predominantly female occupation despite the Sex Discrimination Act (1975) which required restrictions on men practising midwifery to be lifted in 1983. According to NMC statistics (2005) the number of men in midwifery is very low, of the 32,745 midwives who submitted a notification of intention to practise only 115 are men.

The number of shortened midwifery courses for nurses outnumbered the direct entry courses but by the late 1980s nurse recruitment to midwifery was falling and by this time there was only one remaining direct entry midwifery course. The Department of Health provided sufficient funding for seven schools of midwifery to develop direct entry midwifery programmes at diploma level linked to higher education institutions. By 2000 three quarters of midwives had been successfully trained through the direct entry route and this continues.

Midwives welcomed the direct entry route into midwifery but in the long term it may prove problematic for individual midwives in relation to career progression and for the profession as a whole in relation to leadership and management of midwifery services. Maternity services are now inextricably linked to women's health, paediatric and neonatal services and increasingly it is nurses (often without a midwifery qualification) rather than midwives who are in senior NHS management positions and have overall responsibility for midwifery services. That this has become the norm is confirmed in the recently published Shribman Report (DH, 2007) about the proposed reconfiguration of maternity services. Directors of nursing services rather than heads of midwifery services are listed in the target audience for the report.

Anecdotal evidence from NHS Trusts also suggests that direct entry midwives on registration opt to work on a part-time rather than full-time basis. This may be a contributory factor to the ongoing midwifery staffing shortages. NMC statistics (2005) confirm that more than half of practising midwives are working part-time.

Maternity care requires a round the clock service and it may be that because today's students are older, are more likely to have children and may be single parents, that the shift patterns required for full time work is creating child care difficulties that makes full-time work impossible.

A period of full-time practice on registration is desirable because it enables newly qualified midwives to become confident, competent practitioners. Working on a part-time basis does not preclude this but it will take that much longer to achieve. Unlike the nurse entrant, the direct entry student midwife also has to acclimatise to working within the culture of the NHS which may be problematic for some. This is an area in need of research in the interests of both midwives, the future of midwifery and employers.

Comparing Midwife's Role and Activities – Early 20th Century to Early 21st Century

The beginning of the century saw the introduction of the welfare state and social reform was high on the government agenda (similar to today); a further problem was maternal mortality; unlike infant mortality rates which were falling, maternal mortality remained static.

Initially health policies facilitated the midwife to carry out her role and for two decades the role and activities of the midwife expanded. Midwives had greater participation in antenatal classes and after much discussion and debate were permitted to administer pain relief in labour at home.

The 1930s and 1940s saw a reduction in maternal mortality by 50% (Tew, 1995). By the 1950s maternal mortality had fallen even further. This was primarily due to improvement in living conditions and better nutrition but the use of ergometrine and blood transfusion had greatly reduced maternal death due to haemorrhage and the discovery of sulphonamide drugs and penicillin and the use of aseptic techniques virtually eliminated puerperal fever. Whilst this period saw a gradual increase in hospital confinement, midwives remained responsible for the majority of normal pregnancies and births whether at home or in hospital.

But this was not to continue; as the century progressed health care policies began to hinder and often obstruct maximum use of midwifery knowledge and skills because by the 1960s maternal mortality rates had fallen to an all time low, i.e. 0.18 per 1000 births, and the focus of medical attention shifted from maternal mortality to reducing perinatal mortality rates (Donnison, 2004).

Impact of the National Health Service on the Role of the Midwife

The introduction of the NHS in 1948 compounded the problem for midwives because GPs were given a strong incentive to develop antenatal care i.e. a separate fee for midwifery services. Women would also have direct access to GP care independent of the midwife and the obstetrician.

This meant that the first point of contact for pregnant women became the GP rather than the midwife and according to Oakley this 'permanently altered the midwives' control over maternity care' (Oakley, 1986:143). GPs began to see women in early pregnancy giving them, rather than the midwives the opportunity to define normality.

Eventually GPs expanded their role in antenatal care at the expense of the midwife which prompted complaints by Medical Officers of Health and midwives to the Ministry of Health (MOH). The MOH had already set up a working party to investigate the training and terms and conditions of midwives' work because of an apparent shortage of midwives (by 1948 73,613 midwives were on the roll but only 17,095 midwives had notified their intention to practise).

The Report of the Working Party on Midwives (MOH, 1949) acknowledged that general practitioners (GPs) were tending to take over the whole of antenatal care and this was fragmenting midwifery care. The report asked for prompt administrative action by the Ministry of Health to stop what they viewed as an unwelcome trend which could wreck the structure of the midwifery services.

Nonetheless the role of the GP and obstetrician continued to expand and finally in 1980 a report was published which had the greatest impact of all on the kind of maternity care women received and consequently upon the role and activities of the midwife. The Short Report (HMSO, 1980) *Perinatal and Neonatal Mortality* considered that the 'new investigative approach' to maternity care made it inevitable that obstetricians would be required to undertake practices traditionally assigned to the midwife and that included care of 'normal' women. The Short Report was committed to routine use of technology even though:

'...Mothers who have not been adequately prepared may feel that the process of delivery is being dehumanised by technology, and midwives may regret that they are displaced by doctors in the supervision of labour. Nevertheless much of the new technology is of accepted benefit to the mother and baby and we regard it as an integral part of modern maternity care'.

HMSO 1980:72

Furthermore the report made clear that whilst midwives should be given greater responsibility for the care of women with uncomplicated pregnancies the overall supervision of the care of all pregnant women would be:

'...the responsibility of the doctor and we do not consider that midwives should become more active in their role as independent practitioners'

HMSO 1980:72

In response to the recommendations of the Short Report, the Government established a Maternity Services Advisory Committee. Its brief was to address issues surrounding perinatal death rates and ways of improving care for women in maternity hospitals. This resulted in the publication of the Maternity Care in Action Reports, Parts I, II and III (HMSO, 1982, 1984, 1985) as guides to good practice in the maternity services but in reality they exacerbated the problem for midwives by making a clear distinction between antepartum, postpartum and postnatal care which enabled obstetricians to isolate the management of antenatal and intrapartum care from postnatal care which (as in the past) was left to the midwives.

Impact of Technology on Midwifery

By the 1980s ultrasound scanning was integral to antenatal care and investigations and interventions had became so commonplace that they became to be regarded as the norm, for example, antenatal screening, induction and active management of labour supported by continuous electronic fetal heart rate monitoring. Caesarean section rates which had been around 3% in the 1950s would by 2006 have risen to 23% (Shribman, 2007).

By the 1980s midwifery was becoming research based and individual midwives were undertaking research that would demonstrate certain routine midwifery practices were unnecessary for example, pubic shaving (Romney, 1980) and administration of enemas (Romney and Gordon, 1981). Both of these studies contributed to a change in practice. By the end of the century research was integrated into midwifery education and practice and many midwives held research posts.

Growing research awareness meant that whilst midwives accommodated the routine use of technology with many of them perceiving it as an extension of their skills, many midwives were also beginning to challenge the often not research based, routine use of technology, but eventually obstetric practice and routine application of technology to all aspects of the childbearing process became evident in the majority of maternity units which effectively marginalized traditional midwifery practice within the hospital environment (Bates, 1993).

By the 1990s increasingly sophisticated methods of antenatal screening resulted in an increase in fetal medicine and high dependency and neonatal intensive care units proliferated throughout the UK. Patterns of midwifery care were constantly changing to accommodate ongoing reorganisation of maternity services and this took place against a backdrop of increasing litigation and the role and activities of the midwife were subject to a variety of policies, protocols and guidelines and eventually formal risk management standards were implemented in the 1990s.

Impact of Government Policies on Midwifery Practice

By the 1990s government policies were reflecting a drive to reduce obstetric litigation and to provide maternity care that was both clinically and cost effective. The rise in obstetric litigation was due in part to a change in the legal aid rules which were revised in 1990 to enable claims made on behalf of infants to be state funded. There was a UK wide response to this; in England the NHS Litigation Authority (NHSLA) implemented the Clinical Negligence Scheme for Trusts (CNST); The Welsh Risk Pool introduced risk management standards in Wales, and Scotland has the Clinical Negligence and Other Risk Indemnity Scheme (CNORIS) and the Scottish Intercollegiate Guidelines Network (SIGN). Northern Ireland has a Clinical Governance Support Unit. These organisations ensured risk management became integral to maternity care throughout the UK and had a profound impact upon midwifery practice and continues to do so.

Linked to risk management was clinical and cost effectiveness and with this in mind the Audit Commission conducted an audit of maternity care of 2,376 women, 500 GPs and 13 NHS trusts. Their report *A First Class Delivery Service* (Audit Commission, 1997) confirmed a high level of intervention rates and increasing caesarean section rates. The significance of this report is that it was the first document to acknowledge that there were two entirely different philosophies of maternity care, i.e. the traditional midwifery viewpoint that childbirth is normal until it proves itself otherwise as opposed to the medical viewpoint that childbirth can only be normal in retrospect, and each one would result in an entirely different rationale for maternity services. The report recommended that whilst safety should always be of prime concern, maternity care towards the end of the twentieth century should reflect that we are a predominantly healthy nation and in the interests of clinical and cost effectiveness pregnancy and birth should be seen as a normal life event. The nature of the service should be to provide care and support that reflects this view. This report in effect was supporting a traditional midwifery philosophy of care.

However by this time NHS Trusts had introduced management practices that created increasingly stressful demands both within the job itself and the working environment (Ball et al, 2002). Trust managers began implementing government directives to extend the use of specialist midwifery skills and this coincided with continued efforts to reduce employment costs.

Midwives in many units were working longer shifts, had greater workloads and a serious reduction in the number of experienced colleagues. Morale was very low, sickness and turnover rates high (Bates and McNabb, 1996).

In an effort to make 'better use' of midwives the Department of Health published *The Midwifery Action Plan* (DH, 2001) which resulted in an expansion of the midwives role to include tasks previously confined to doctors such as examination of the newborn. This was further developed to include some midwives undertaking breech, ventouse and forceps deliveries and gaining an ultrasound qualification.

Midwives also began to work within programmes such as Sure Start that was set up in response to concern about a lack of parenting skills. Traditionally preparation for parenting was integral to the role of the midwife but it too had become a casualty of the medicalisation of childbearing as the focus of antenatal classes became preparation for labour which had become quite complex. It could be argued that in the interests of public health and social reform the role of the midwife was becoming ill defined.

Autonomous Midwifery Practice

The passing of the Midwives Act in 1902 legitimised midwifery practice but the Act required the newly appointed Central Midwives Board to produce a framework of midwives rules to regulate the training and practice of midwives, set examinations and keep a roll of registered midwives (Myles, 1964) and understandably the independent midwives at the time perceived this as a loss of autonomy.

Subsequent regulatory bodies have periodically updated the Midwives rules and the current Midwives rules and standards, Rule 6: Responsibility and sphere of practice states that a midwife is accountable for her own practice and yet the guidance within Rule 6 also states that: '...practice must be based upon locally agreed evidence based standards...' (NMC, 2004:18). This guidance is open to interpretation but it implies the midwife is not an autonomous practitioner.

Initially midwives worked with a considerable degree of autonomy retaining much of their traditional control over childbearing. Opportunities for independent practice continued to exist but further legislation in 1936 completed the transition from independent midwifery practice to state salaried employment for the majority of midwives.

By the time the NHS was introduced in 1948, obstetrics had become established as a separate discipline and GPs became integral to the provision of maternity care. This began the erosion of midwifery autonomy in earnest; for example, making the GP the first point of contact for all pregnant women, and the gradual shift from home to hospital confinement. As the century progressed scientific knowledge advanced and childbirth became institutionalized. Obstetrics became the dominant discourse. It culminated in the publication of the Short Report, Perinatal and Neonatal Mortality (HMSO, 1980) which finally ended midwifery autonomy by handing over responsibility for the care of all pregnant women to the obstetrician. This fundamentally changed the role of the midwife.

The Short report also displayed a profound change in attitude towards women and they too lost their autonomy. Previous reports had been sensitive to women's preferences, whereas the Short Report dismissed the preferences of women as irrelevant to policy formulation because women's preferences were seen as incompatible with the medical determination of risk (Oakley, 1986).

The publication of *Changing Childbirth* (DH, 1993) in England brought back the potential for a degree of autonomous midwifery practice by giving women a choice of lead professional and choice in place of birth. But at the same time risk assessment and management practices were gathering apace and the implementation of formal risk management standards/guidelines for maternity care throughout the UK further eroded the notion of autonomous midwifery practice.

Kirkham highlighted a culture of midwifery in the NHS that made uncomfortable reading (Kirkham, 1999). Research funded by the Royal College of Midwives, *Why Midwives Leave?*, highlighted the many problems for midwives working in the NHS that probably contributed to this culture. Midwives felt they had very little, if any control over the way they practised and this had resulted in many of them deciding to leave midwifery practice (Ball et al, 2002).

Birth Centres appear to offer midwives the opportunity for a degree of autonomous practice but these are under threat. A reconfiguration of the maternity services is planned which could result in extremely large consultant led maternity units (Shribman, 2007) and the potential for closure of midwife led units.

Over the years the medical profession has contributed to the good health of mothers and babies and women with complicated pregnancies need their expertise; but insisting that all women should be considered at risk until they had given birth and proven otherwise has not been helpful to fit, healthy women with uncomplicated pregnancies, who appear to have lost confidence in their ability to give birth without some form of intervention and it has resulted in an increase in maternal morbidity (MacArthur et al, 1991; Bick and MacArthur, 1995)

It has also contributed to the culture of midwifery in the NHS as described by Kirkham (1999). This is the result of the steady erosion of autonomous midwifery practice over many decades that has restricted the options available to women, marginalized midwifery practice and promoted childbearing as a pathological medicalised process (Oakley and Houd, 1990).

Midwifery in the 21st Century

The history of midwifery is one of struggle and the continuing problems for midwifery in the NHS since its inception have been well documented (Oakley, 1976; Oakley, 1980; 1986, 1993; Donnison, 1988; Oakley and Houd, 1990; Bates, 1993; Kirkham, 1999; Ball et al, 2002; Bates, 2004).

It could be argued that NHS policies and management practices do not allow midwives to fulfil their potential as professionals and the challenge for midwives in the 21st century will be to find ways of taking ownership of research based midwifery skills and knowledge and maintaining their clinical expertise to support the psychological, emotional and physiological processes of pregnancy, labour and birth along with the appropriate use of technology.

It has always been integral to the role of the midwife to find ways of opening up options for women regardless of risk and to assist them to develop an internal locus of control to promote self confidence and self esteem to sustain them during labour and birth and the early weeks of motherhood. The need for these fundamental midwifery skills remains essential to the wellbeing of mothers and babies in the 21st century.

Activity 8

1. What skills do you think a midwife needs to meet the needs of pregnant women?

2. Explore ways in which midwives can assist women to become self-confident about the childbearing process.

3. How can midwives help couples develop their parenting skills during pregnancy?

4. What do you think are the reasons for the increase in postnatal depression rates in recent years?

References

Audit Commission (1997) *First Class Delivery: improving maternity services in England and Wales.* Audit Commission, London

Ball L, Curtis P, Kirkham M (2002) *Why do midwives leave?* Royal College of Midwives, London

Bates C (1993) Care in normal labour: a feminist perspective In: Alexander J. Levy V, Roth C eds. *Midwifery Practice: Core Topics 2.* Macmillan Press Ltd, London

Bates C, McNabb M (1996) Governing midwifery practice. *British Journal of Midwifery* **4**(3): 119–20

Bates C (2004) Midwifery practice and ways of working. In: Stewart M. *Pregnancy, Birth and Maternity Care: feminist perspectives.* Elsevier Science Ltd, London

Bewley S, Friend J, Mezey G (eds) (1997) *Violence against women.* RCOG Press, London

Bick DE, MacArthur C (1995) The extent, severity and effect of health problems after childbirth. *British Journal of Midwifery* **3**(1): 27–31

Chambers R, Wakley G, Chambers S (2001) *Tackling teenage pregnancy: Sex, culture and needs.* Radcliffe Medical Press, Abingdon

Cranbrook Report: Report of the Maternity Services Committee (1959) HMSO, London

Dennison C (2004) *Teenage Pregnancy: an overview of the research evidence.* Health Development Agency, Wetherby

Department of Health and Social Security Welsh Office Standing Maternity And Midwifery Advisory Committee (1970) *Domiciliary midwifery and maternity bed needs report of the Sub- Committee.* HMSO, London

Briggs A, Chairman (1972) *Report of the Committee on Nursing* (Cmnd 5115). HMSO, London

DH (1993) *Changing Childbirth: Report of the Expert Maternity Group.* HMSO, London

Northern Ireland Maternity Unit Study Group (1994) *Delivering Choice: midwife and general practitioner led maternity units.* DHSS, Belfast

DH (1996) *The patients charter maternity services.* Department of Health, London

DH (1999) *Saving Lives. Our Healthier Nation.* Stationery Office, London

DH (2001a) *Tackling Health Inequalities Consultation on a Plan for Delivery.* Department of Health, London

DH (2001b) *Midwifery action plan: "Making a difference – the nursing, midwifery and health visiting contribution."* DoH, Leeds

Donnison J In Henderson C Macdonald S (Eds) (2004) Mayes' a Textbook for Midwives, 13th edn. Baillière Tindall, Edinburgh

House of Commons (1980) Second Report from the Social Services Committee Session 1979-1980, Perinatal and Neonatal Mortality, Vol.1. HMSO, London

House of Commons Health Committee (1992) Maternity Services: Health Committee, second report. (Chairman Nicholas Winterton). Vol 1 Report together with appendices and the proceedings of the committee. HMSO, London

Kirkham M (1999) The culture of midwifery in the National Health Service in England. *Journal of Advanced Nursing* **30**(3): 732–9

Klaus MH, Kennell JH (1976) *Maternal - Infant Bonding.* Mosby, St Louis

MacArthur C, Lewis M, Knox EG (1991) *Health after Childbirth.* HMSO, London

Maternity Services Advisory Committee (1982) Maternity care in action. Part 1 Antenatal care. A guide to good practice and a plan for action. First report. HMSO, London

Ministry of Health, Department of Health for Scotland, Ministry of Labour and national Service (1949) The Report of the Working Party on Midwives. HMSO, London

Ministry of Health (1959) Report of the Maternity Services Committee (Cranbrook). HMSO, London

Myles MF (1964) *A Textbook for Midwives* 5th edn. E & S Livingstone Ltd, Edinburgh and London

Nursing and Midwifery Council (2004) *Midwives rules and standards.* NMC, London

Nursing and Midwifery Council National (2005) Statistics of the Register 1 April 2004 to 31 March 2005 new stats due end of March 2007 would like to include them

Oakley A (1972) *Sex, Gender and Society.* Maurice Temple Smith Ltd, London

Oakley A. Wisewoman and medicine man in Mitchell J. Oakley A. (Eds) (1976) The Rights and Wrongs of Women, Pelican Books, London

Oakley A (1980) *Women Confined: Towards sociology of childbirth.* Martin Robertson, Oxford

Oakley A (1986) *The Captured Womb: A History of the Medical Care of Pregnant Women.* Basil Blackwood Ltd, Oxford

Oakley A (1987) The family in crisis The woman's place. *New Society* **79**(6): 14–16

Oakley A, Houd S (1990) Helpers in Childbirth: Midwifery Today, Hemisphere Pub, New York

Oakley A (1992) The changing social context of pregnancy care. In: Zander L, Chamberlain G eds. *Pregnancy Care in the 1990s.* Parthenon Publishing group, Lancs, England

Oakley A (1993) Essays on Women, Medicine & Health, Edinburgh University Press

Oakley A, Mitchell J (eds) (1997) *Who's Afraid of Feminism? Seeing Through the Backlash.* Penguin, London, London

O'Hara MW, Swain AM (1996) Rates and risks of postpartum depression: a meta-analysis. *International Review of Psychiatry* **8:** 37–54

Royal College of Midwives (2004) *Student Midwives Hardship Campaign Pack.* RCM, London

Romney ML, Gordon H (1981) is your enema really necessary? *British Medical Journal* **282**(6272): 1269–71

Sandall J (1996) Moving towards caseload practice: what evidence do we have? *British Journal of Midwifery* **4**(12): 620–1

Sandall J (1999) Team midwifery and burnout in midwives in the UK: practical lessons from a national study. *MIDIRs Midwifery Digest* **9**(2) 147–52

Scottish Office (1993) *Provision of Maternity Services in Scotland: A Policy Review.* HMSO, Edinburgh?

Shribman S (2007) *Making it Better: For Mother and Baby.* Department of Health, London,

Tew M (1995) *Safer Childbirth? A Critical History of Maternity Care.* 2nd eds. Chapman & Hall, London

Welsh Office (1991) Protocol for Investment in health gain: maternal and early child health

CHAPTER 9

Feminist Perspectives in Midwifery

Carol Bates

Throughout the 20th century, technology and the impact of the feminist movement profoundly changed the lives of women and men both in the home and in the workplace but despite midwifery being a primarily female occupation midwives as a group have yet to embrace feminism. This is puzzling because women have long been subjected to a masculine (obstetric) view of birth which as scientific knowledge advanced has had a profound impact on the nature of maternity care and the organisation of maternity services, both of which have had an equally profound impact on the role and activities of the midwife. Feminism explored the role and position of women in society and offered an alternative way of interpreting the social world. Eventually many different aspects of feminism emerged and consequently feminist scholarship is wide ranging.

Whilst the influence of feminism improved the overall position of women in society the same cannot be said for midwives as a group. Our status did not improve because the sophisticated nature of technology relating to all aspects of fertility ensured that obstetrics remained the dominant discourse and initially feminism did not help midwives. The early feminists were more focussed on getting women into the medical profession from which they were excluded and consequently the plight of the midwives who were struggling for survival was overlooked. It was the radical feminists in the 1970s and 1980s who unwittingly came to the aid of midwifery when they began to write prolifically about the medical control of childbirth, for example Mitchell and Oakley (1976), Rich (1977), Ehrenreich and English (1979), Oakley (1980,1986, 1993) Oakley and Houd (1990).

Feminism explored the role and position of women in society and offered an alternative way of interpreting the social world. Eventually many different aspects of feminism emerged and consequently feminist scholarship is wide ranging for example, there are liberal feminists' who sought property and voting rights and freedom of speech for women. Marxist feminists' explored, political, social and economic structures whilst radical feminists focussed upon reproduction, mothering, gender and sexuality. There is also psychoanalytic feminism which rejected many of Freud's theories especially the Oedipus complex and the notion of penis envy and instead reinterpreted Freudian theory to focus upon the strengths of being a woman and the importance of the early mother-infant relationship (Chodorow, 1978; Dinnerstein, 1987).

Despite midwifery's apparent reluctance to engage with feminism, feminist thinking is a powerful resource for midwifery practice and it is difficult to understand why it continues to be largely overlooked by midwives who spend their working lives with women; feminism offers an insight into the social structures and underlying forces that shape women's lives and for this reason alone it is worth exploring.

Feminism in the UK

The 'first wave' of feminism in the UK began at the turn of the 20th century when British women joined the Women's Suffrage movement and campaigned relentlessly until women won the right to vote. This was a hard fought campaign because opponents of votes for women were afraid that giving women a political voice would fundamentally change the traditional relationship between men and women in the family (Hannam, 2007). Two World Wars were also to dramatically change women's lives because it gave women the opportunity to do paid work customarily carried out by men. At the end of the war women were expected to return to domesticity but they were reluctant to do so because their horizons had widened and they had developed skills in the workplace for which they had been paid.

Despite recognition of the women's war effort, post war propaganda urged women to return to the hearth and home and men to return to work but fortunately the needs of the economy along with the need to rebuild the fabric of post war British society brought about a change in government attitude towards women and work.

But whilst women were actively encouraged to work they did not do so on equal terms with men and by the 1960s the 'second wave' of feminism began seeking equality for women both in the home and in the workplace. The initial focus of second wave feminism was equal pay for equal work, fertility, housework and childcare. Later on the focus included male power, sexual identity and gender violence. Eventually legislation such as equal pay, sex discrimination laws, the Abortion Act and finally making domestic violence a criminal offence (Bewley et al, 1997) improved the lives of women in society.

Initially the second wave feminists were usually white, educated, middle class and heterosexual, but as differences in women based on class, race and sexual orientation began to surface so did the divisions within feminism. Working class women were not drawn to feminism and lesbian feminists obviously had an entirely different agenda. Black women could not agree with their white sisters that sexism was more oppressive than racism and pursued their own theories about gender and race.

Consequently feminist thinking may appear fragmented but there was a common thread that linked them all; an agreement that the root cause of women's suppression and oppression in society was patriarchy (male power and superiority) which feminism considered was sustained and maintained through clearly defined gender roles in society.

Gender Roles

Because of their childbearing and child rearing role women were considered to be the weaker and therefore inferior sex. Marriage rendered women subservient to their husbands and the emphasis for women was their domestic role and family life. Gender roles both in the home and the workplace were clearly defined and this profoundly affected the status of women in society. Gender roles were brought into sharp relief by the second wave of feminism in the 1970s. Feminists argued that discrimination against women was embedded in the ways in which gender roles of men and women, and the meaning of masculinity and femininity were constructed in the media and advertising and everyday language.

The reasons why gender influences remain and women are still not on equal terms with men in the workplace (or in the home) are deep rooted and complex and this chapter does not have the space to address them all but the underlying cause is patriarchy. As barriers were broken down in the 1970s and women entered the public sphere patriarchal values became less apparent, but they simmer under the surface and patriarchy remains pervasive in society.

Consequently women continue to be discriminated against. Women may be present in the workplace and in many institutions but not on equal terms with men because they are subordinated within them (Figes, 1995; Oakley and Mitchell, 1997) and often it will be other women perpetuating the inequality. The feminist philosopher Bartky suggested that this situation arises when women have 'a divided consciousness'. Women may be aware they are victims of an unjust system of power but they perceive it as being natural and consequently unwittingly subscribe to it (Bartky 1990).

Patriarchy

Feminists have argued for decades that it was the all pervasive nature and power of patriarchy that enabled gender inequality to be maintained for so long (Oakley, 1972; Rich, 1977; Walby, 1990). Kate Millett's influential book *Sexual Politics* (1969) argued powerfully that patriarchy underpinned all social constructs including the family, religion, the law and the workplace.

Midwifery's struggle for survival over many centuries demonstrates the all pervasive nature and power of patriarchy and how it enabled gender inequality to be maintained. Adrienne Rich, a radical feminist from the 1970s, gave an all-embracing definition of patriarchy. She described it as:

> *'A familial-social, ideological, political system in which men – by force, direct pressure, or through ritual, tradition, law and language, customs, etiquette, education, and the division of labour, determine what part women shall or shall not play, and in which the female is everywhere subsumed under the male'.*

Rich, 1977

This description could be applied to a consultant-led unit there are rituals and customs, policies and guidelines that direct midwifery practice and a clear division of labour that determines the role and activities of the midwife. This enables obstetric practice to control two groups of women, pregnant women and midwives, and has contributed to the culture of midwifery in the NHS as described by Kirkham (1999). The behaviour she describes is that of an oppressed group and eventually the oppressed become their own oppressors (Bartky, 1998).

Walby (1990) considered patriarchy to have both a private and a public sphere. Private patriarchy was based on gender inequalities in the home and public patriarchy based on inequality and discrimination in public life. Society is now more complex in relation to class, culture, race, age, and ethnicity and there are different kinds of femininities and masculinities but the concept of patriarchy remains useful for shedding light on gender inequalities if the complexities of society are taken into consideration (Pilcher, 1998).

The medical profession is a powerful patriarchal institution and this continued well into the late 20th century despite increasing numbers of women entering the medical profession (Elston, 1993). The problem for women entering a predominantly male discipline such as obstetrics is that collectively this group will express a masculine view of childbirth and to be successful the women need to subscribe to this view and according to Hicks study (1991) they do this very successfully because midwives consider obstetricians regardless of sex to be superior to midwives. In contrast midwifery has remained a predominantly female occupation and consequently without the status and therefore power of the medical profession.

Midwives have attempted to challenge patriarchy in its various forms, initially the Church and then the medical profession and now the state.

We have not been successful and consequently the patriarchal control of childbearing has been well documented by feminist writers (Rich, 1977; Ehrenreich and English, 1979; Oakley, 1976, 1980, 1986, 1993).

Towards the end of the 20th century the medical profession was no longer the prime source of patriarchal power. Whilst still powerful, it did not exercise the same degree of power as in the past. The reorganisation of the NHS in the early 1990s gave greater power to other sources of patriarchy power, for example general managers and chief executives of trusts and the legal profession.

A powerful driver for change in 1990 was the revision of the legal aid rules. From hereon all claims on behalf of infants became state funded (Hardman and Bates, 2005). Inevitably this boosted the number of claims. The ensuing fear of litigation and the cost to the NHS made it equally inevitable that a more formal approach to risk assessment and management would be adopted.

Huge expenditure on clinical negligence claims led to the setting up of the NHS Litigation Authority and implementation of the Clinical Negligence Scheme for Trusts (CNST) in 1994. This has led to defensive practice by both midwives and obstetricians and has further eroded the role of the midwife. The legal profession had become a potent source of patriarchal power within the maternity services.

The recently published Shribman Report *Making It Better: For Mother and Baby* (DH, 2007) states the case for replacing local maternity units with large regional maternity centres whilst retaining midwife led units and the choice of home birth. But the report highlights that only 2-3% of babies are born at home and only 4% of babies are born in a midwife led birthing centre. This means that eventually midwife led units and home birth facilities could well be withdrawn. Funding is a critical issue for the NHS; with such small numbers involved, in the event of further financial crisis closure of a midwife led unit or withdrawal of home birth facilities will be seen as the most cost effective action to take. This will once again give obstetricians overall control of childbearing and enable the return of patriarchal power.

If midwives choose not to work in them, they will be replaced by maternity care assistants. Some trusts are already meeting the shortfall of midwives by employing maternity care assistants and it could be argued that maternity care assistants are a potential threat to the future of midwifery practice.

Economic Bondage

This remains a huge issue for many women. Whilst the days when the man was the bread winner and supported his wife and family may be long gone, women in the 21st century remain subject to economic bondage. Women often seek part-time work to supplement the family income and because family responsibilities have priority over work , even though the money earned might be vital to the family remaining solvent, the lack of affordable childcare meant work had to be part-time and was therefore likely to be low skilled and low paid.

Eyer (1992) placed the blame for this thinking about women and work on male theories about pregnancy, birth, breastfeeding and maternal infant bonding, e.g. Bowlby (1958), Klaus and Kennel (1976), which were used to justify women being seen as the 'natural' carers of very young children and according to Oakley (1972) this view underpinned the gendered division of labour in the home and the workplace. This belief exists in many cultures in the UK today.

The Equal Pay Act (1970) and the Sex Discrimination Act (1975) were meant to restrict discrimination on grounds of sex and reduce the gender gap in earnings. But Figes (1995) maintained that this legislation gave women a sense of false security because discrimination against women continued but went virtually unnoticed. Employment patterns for decades were based on systems biased towards men's working patterns i.e. uninterrupted, full time work which meant that women, who were more likely to be in part-time work because of domestic responsibilities and childcare, could never hope to gain parity with men.

Times have changed and many women work full-time and some women have reached highly paid executive positions in the city, are lawyers and hospital consultants. At the other end of the scale are poorly educated, unemployed single mothers living on welfare. Single, unemployed parents are being encouraged to work through the *New Deal for Lone Parents* initiative, a voluntary programme specifically designed to help lone parents (usually mothers) into work.

In the middle is a vast army of women (this includes midwives) with average incomes struggling to juggle work and family commitments. There is a lack of affordable childcare and much of the earnings of these women go towards paying for childcare. Women now have two roles; they labour for money at work and labour for love at home. Legislation has attempted to improve this situation by introducing flexible working rights in 2003 and The Work and Families Act (2006) extended this to include the carers of adults which, like child care is usually the responsibility of women.

There is also a very large group of women who are rarely mentioned, the women who work from home doing typing or sewing, taking in ironing or filling hundreds of envelopes. These women are the most disadvantaged of all. The rates of pay are very low, they provide their own equipment and there are no fringe benefits. Many of these women are well qualified but see this work as a stop gap whilst children are very small.

The problem is a gender pay gap persists and having children continues to affect women's job prospects, consequently women are still over represented in part-time, low skilled low paid work. Lower-paid jobs are also less likely to have occupational pension schemes.

This came about because patriarchal institutions rather than encouraging child welfare to become the concern of both men and women influenced government policies to ensure that child care remained a woman and work issue. This was the price women had to pay if they wanted to have children and work.

This attitude was exacerbated by women in influential positions in both large organisations and government. They had made it to the top but were not inclined to assist their less influential sisters to take control of their lives. They were more likely to press for social welfare reform than gender equality in the home and workplace.

The report of the *Women and Work Commission, Shaping a Fairer Future* (DTI, 2006) offers hope for the future. It acknowledges that the issues around women and work puts women at an unfair disadvantage because their lower earnings leave them at greater risk of falling below the poverty line and of being worse off than men in retirement.

The report also confirms gender stereotyping remains. Choices about work are still affected by deep rooted assumptions about the abilities and attributes of men and women and concludes that a culture change is needed in order to challenge assumptions about the types of jobs women and men can do. This is likely to take time but is essential if the gender pay gap is to be resolved and women are to be released from economic bondage.

Feminist Backlash

Towards the end of the 20th century a backlash against feminism began. Feminism began to be blamed for many of society's ills especially the breakdown in family life (Oakley, 1987; French, 1992; Oakley and Mitchell, 1997). At the root of the backlash was a fear of feminism similar to the fears expressed when women were seeking the right to vote. Oakley and Mitchell (1997) considered the backlash was also recognition of the power of feminism to change women's lives. For Faludi the basis of the backlash was a desire to systematically undermine women and their progress in society (Faludi, 1992).

Coward (1999) contributed to the feminist backlash and gives a good example of fear of feminism when she argues that feminism had demonized men and damaged relations between men and women. If Coward is right in her assumptions about the effects of feminism, the underlying cause will not be feminism but the reluctance on the part of men (and some women) to accept that women have a right to equality.

The problem for society is not feminism but patriarchy, which rather than help women to achieve equality, has consistently and systematically moved the goal posts to hamper women's progress in society (Faludi, 1992; French, 1992; Oakley and Mitchell, 1997).

A Third Wave of Feminism?

The media (a powerful patriarchal institution) coined the phrase post feminism to imply that feminism was no longer relevant to society. So is there a place for feminism in the 21st century?

Whilst many women have taken full advantage of the educational, employment and reproductive rights that feminism made possible, not all women have benefited from these social and economic changes. Women as a group still do not have equality, the gender pay gap persists and too many women and children live below the poverty line.

There is at present in the UK the political will, albeit in the interests of the British economy, to reduce gender influences in the workplace but child welfare remains problematic and this according to UNICEF is because of economic inequality and poor levels of public support for families in the UK (UNICEF, 2006). The UK is also now a multicultural society and deep rooted private patriarchy persists in many cultures.

The United Nations Children's Fund (UNICEF) report *The State of the World's Children 2007: Women and Children the Double Dividend of Gender Equality* (UNICEF 2006) is about the lives of women and children around the world. The report concluded that gender equality and the well-being of children go hand in hand. When women are empowered to live full and productive lives, children prosper but if women are denied equal opportunity within a society then children suffer. This report demonstrates that feminism was not just about women and men can be feminists too.

The feminist movement gained momentum during the 20th century reflecting the needs of women at the time. A feminist consciousness cannot be given to women, they must discover it for themselves and the life experience of women in the 21st century will eventually define feminism for them. Women are already involved in human rights and environmentalism; political and economic globalisation could bring a third wave of feminism that sees men and women joining together across national boundaries to enable sustained action against common forms of oppression of women that persist around the world. But will midwives participate? Hopefully they will because if midwives were to develop a feminist consciousness this would be a bonus for the profession and for women. As Kaufmann (2004) points out a feminist midwife understands the meaning of power and powerlessness and how this shapes women's experiences as maternity service users as well as midwives' experiences as workers in the service. Ultimately, feminist midwifery profession would maximize the autonomy of both women and midwives.

Activity 9

1. What are your views about the impact of feminism on society?

2. Think about how government policies affect midwifery practice and the care women receive.

3. To what extent does obstetric practice affect midwifery practice on the labour ward?

3. Do pregnant women have autonomy?

References

Bartky SL (1990) *Femininity and domination: studies in the phenomenology of oppression.* Routledge, London

Bartky SL (1998) On Psychological Oppression. In: Rogers MF, ed. *Contemporary Feminist Theory.* McGraw Hill

Bewley S, Friend F, Mezey G (1997) *Violence against women.* RCOG Press, London

Bowlby J (1953) *Child Care and the Growth of Love.* Harmondsworth Penguin, London

Chodorow N (1978) *The Reproduction of Mothering: Psychoanalysis and the Sociology of Gender.* University of California Press, London

Coward R (1999) *Sacred Cows: Is Feminism Relevant to the New Millennium?* Harper Collins Publishers, London

Dinnerstein D (1987) *The rocking of the cradle the ruling of the world.* The Women's Press Ltd, London

Elston MA (1993) In: Riska E, Wegar K, eds. *Gender, Work and Medicine.* Sage Publications Ltd, London

Ehrenreich B, English D (1979) *For her own good.* Pluto Press, London

Eyer DE (1992) *Mother-Infant Bonding a Scientific Fiction.* Yale University

Figes K (1995) *Because of her sex: The Myth of Equality for Women in Britain*. Pan Books, London

Faludi S. (1992) *Backlash: The Undeclared War Against Women*. Chatto & Windus Ltd, London

French M (1992) *The War Against Women*. Penguin Books, London

Hannam J (2007) *Feminism*. Pearson Education Ltd

Hardman L, Bates C (2005) *Litigation: a risk management guide for midwives*. Royal College of Midwives and Capsticks Solicitors London second edition

Kaufmann T (2004) In: Stewart M, ed. *Pregnancy, Birth and Maternity Care: a feminist perspective*. Books for Midwives, London

Kirkham M (1999) The culture of midwifery in the National Health Service in England *Journal of Advanced Nursing* **30**(3): 732-739

Klaus MH, Kennell JH (1976) *Maternal - Infant Bonding*. St Louis Mosby

Millett K (1969) *Sexual Politics* Rupert Hart Davis

Oakley A (1972) *Sex, Gender and Society*. Maurice Temple Smith Ltd, London

Oakley A (1976) Wisewoman and medicine man. In: Mitchell J, Oakley A, eds. *The Rights and Wrongs of Women*. Pelican Books, London

Oakley A (1980) *Women Confined* Martin Robertson, Oxford

Oakley A (1986) *The Captured Womb: A History of the Medical Care of Pregnant Women*. Basil Blackwood Ltd, Oxford

Oakley A (1987) *The family in crisis. The woman's place*. New Society, March, 79 (6): 14-16

Oakley A, Houd S (1990) *Helpers in Childbirth: Midwifery Today, London Hemisphere on behalf of WHO regional office for Europe*. WHO, Geneva

Oakley A (1993) *Essays on Women, Medicine and Health*. Edinburgh University Press

Oakley A, Mitchell J eds (1997) *Who's Afraid of Feminism? Seeing Through the Backlash*. Hamish Hamilton, London

Pilcher R (1998) Hormones of hegemonic masculinity? Explaining gender and gender inequalities. *Sociology Review* February 5-9

Rich A (1977) *Of woman born: motherhood as experience and institution*. Virago London

Shribman S (2007) *Making it Better: For Mother and Baby*. Department of Health, London

The United Nations Children's Fund (UNICEF) (2006) *The State of the World's Children 2007: Women and Children the Double Dividend of Gender Equality* UNICEF (December)

Walby S (1990) *Theorizing Patriarchy*. Basil Blackwood Ltd, Oxford

Women & Work Commission (2006) *Shaping a Fairer Future*. Department of Trade and Industry (February) DTI/Pub 8057/5.0k/02/06/NP. URN 06/697

CHAPTER 10

Conflict, Culture and Opportunities for Midwives

Sue Jacob

'The best year the NHS has had'
> Patricia Hewitt Secretary of State for Health 2006

The above statement by Patricia Hewitt sent the media into a frenzy of highlighting the inadequacy of the National Health Service (NHS) in meeting the public demand and expectations of health care service. Healthcare clinicians assert that whilst the NHS reforms are welcome, some of them are unworkable. This chapter identifies aspects of the NHS reforms and modernization agenda that impact on midwifery and midwives and aims to raise student midwives' awareness of the range of factors that influence the provision of maternity services and the midwife's role. It concludes with strategies for midwives to survive or overcome the contradictions.

Context for Conflict

There is a consensus amongst conflict theorists that the defining characteristic of conflict is inequality, and that the most powerful or dominant groups socialise the least powerful into accepting inequality. Hyman (1975) argues that conflict is inevitable between the employee and the employer as each group's priorities and interests are different. The employer is concerned with productivity and profits, while the employee is often concerned with quality of relationships and the remuneration of his effort.

Kirkham (2006) identifies the contradictions experienced by the midwives in their roles as employees and as professionals. They experience stress and conflict when their relationship with women was compromised by inadequate resources and were powerless to influence their circumstances. The current climate of budget deficits is also affecting midwifery staffing levels, which in turn are impacting on provision of services. In some cases the services are being cut and staff have been made redundant (Manero, 2003), thus compromising the type of care the women/users want or require.

The tendency to rationalise, reconfigure, merge services and adopt a 'one size fits all' philosophy appears to dominate service delivery, thereby further exacerbating staff morale and job satisfaction (Bosanquet, 2005).

The modernisation agenda of healthcare professionals' careers is introducing a wide range of roles that are unregulated and yet deployed to deliver direct care (NHS Employers, 2006; Sandall, 2007). This creates a potential to not only fragment and substitute existing professional roles but also affect the foundations of quality care, for example continuity of care, accountability, building of trusting relationships with the users of care and protection of the public.

NHS Ideology

As the NHS transforms itself from a monolithic organisation to a system of pluralist providers of health care, it is inevitable that conflict/tension is likely to occur between the competing providers. Whilst the four countries are committed to maintaining the principle of UK NHS, the *New NHS: Modern and Dependable* (DH, 1997) maintains the principle of a national health service with an emphasis on modernisation. The modernisation agenda is structured around themes of clinical governance, a flexible workforce, user involvement and addressing inequalities. *The NHS Plan: A plan for investment, A plan for reform* (DH, 2000; Scottish Executive, 2000; National Assembly for Wales, 2001) set a 10-year vision and direction for the implementation of the modernisation agenda. The pace of reforms and ideology in all four countries in the UK are transforming the way we think about the health service and the way care is delivered.

Whilst progress is being made in developing a service that is responsive to the needs of local population, including user involvement and introducing systems to develop a skilled workforce (DH, 2004a) in order to meet the demands and expectations of the users, a centrally-driven target culture is detracting the local providers from addressing the health priorities of the local population. For example, the national target of reducing waiting times is detracting the managers from setting local priorities and diverting resources away from maternity services.

The NHS reforms of the 1990s (DH, 1997, 1998, 2000; Scottish Executive, 2000; National Assembly for Wales, 2001) signpost a fundamental shift in the ideology of a publicly-funded health service. The notion of a centralised monopoly for provision of services is rejected in favour of a pluralist system. As the cost of healthcare provision escalates, the ideology of a nationally funded public service is shifting towards the creation of a pluralist model of health service with multiple stakeholders, for example independent with vested commercial and capitalist interests, voluntary sectors with social responsibility, and more recently a social enterprise model that seeks to overcome barriers of bureaucracy and provide an alternative model of care.

The government's vision of 'commissioning a patient-led service' (Crisp, 2005) reinforces the notion of a greater use of diverse providers whilst strengthening the commissioning role at strategic health authority and health board levels. The plurality of providers from voluntary, independent and social sectors offers options and choices in care at primary, secondary and tertiary levels in alternative settings thereby deconstructing the dominance and monopoly of care delivery in the NHS acute sector. The deployment of a plurality of providers within maternity services offers a scope for shifting the focus of provision of care from acute sector to community, thus promoting and enhancing 'well-being' instead of a 'sickness care' model in childbirth. However, the use of a plurality of providers presents potential risks of creating a two-tier care system and inadequate systems in financing, auditing and monitoring of care standards within the independent and voluntary sectors presents a challenge.

The White Paper *Our Health, Our Care, Our Say* (DH, 2006) sets a direction for developing and strengthening services in a community that best fit the local population needs. Whilst involving the community in planning and making decisions about their local health care provision, healthcare professionals are being encouraged to develop new ways of working by engaging in a social enterprise model (Lewis et al, 2006).

Social Enterprise Model

The social enterprise model aims to allow professionals to become partners in care delivery, for example it offers midwives the opportunity to exercise full scope of their role, become self-employed, work in partnership with general practitioners, develop innovative partnership working models and create a financially viable business unit.

Although the social enterprise model appears favourable and offers an opportunity to midwives, there are challenges in setting up infrastructure for appropriate care delivery, lines and systems for accountability for adverse clinical incidents, the position and status of midwives in new partnership models and the establishment of risk management system. The independent midwifery model has been cited as offering a scope to advance the social entrepreneurship model in midwifery. For midwives to engage in a plurality of provision, NHS vicarious liability systems at national level will need to develop an inclusive system to harness the requirements of professionals providing care through diverse models. We need to consider the financial impact of social enterprise model on clinical placement experience for student midwives as the practitioners in the business unit will require remuneration for their services.

Payment By Results

The NHS financial reforms articulated in *Delivering the NHS Plan* link payment to clinical activity known as 'payment by results' (PBR) (DH, 2007c). This creates an establishment of agreed tariffs across the NHS for particular clinical activity to promote transparency and fairness.

The prevalence of a bio-medical model and risk management culture attracts funding for mandatory training as part of risk management for clinical negligence schemes, whilst resources for midwifery professional development are difficult to access. Lack of resources for supporting midwives in providing holistic care models is alienating midwives from their core activities and midwifery skills. The 'soft' aspects of clinical activity are not awarded a payment tariff. Some of the core activities performed by midwives are at variance with price tariffs: for example home deliveries, community midwifery and clinics where a medical consultant is not present are not within the PBR scope.

The PBR scheme is expected to reward providers with high productivity. However, when providers are incentivised by payment per activity there is a tendency to increase the pace of activity, creating a conveyer belt ethos and thus compromising the quality. Although the payment by results system of economic accountability is commendable in ensuring transparency, it has the potential to create competition and tension between clinicians' autonomy and professional standards in clinical activity and managers' desire to increase clinical productivity.

Additionally, normal birth costs less than one with interventions, hence PBR appears discriminatory towards midwives' role and clinical activities. Midwives express frustration with PBR, as it does not value their professional practice — that which underpins their ability to deliver woman centred holistic care and offer choices for options of care models.

It could be argued that PBR scheme could undermine the viability of birth centres and midwifery-led care units — where the numbers of women giving birth continue to remain small.

Culture of the NHS

The notion of culture of an organisation remains an elusive concept; however there is a consensus on the elements that constitute culture in health services, for example, shared values, beliefs and attitudes between colleagues. The NHS comprises different groups of professionals, each with its own subculture. Davies et al (2000) identify three elements — assumptions, values and artefacts — from which each subculture takes its identity. The dominance of any particular subculture depends on the power and influence it exerts within the organisation.

The power and influence exerted by midwives appears to be limited. Kirkham (1999) highlights that the midwives experience helplessness and they often operate in an environment that does not 'value them as women'. They perceive any support offered as 'policing and controlling' rather than as genuine care and interest. She also suggests that there is a lack of role models in a culture of 'sacrifice, service, guilt and blame', and that midwives feel frustrated at a forked-tongue approach to care delivery: on the one hand there is a desire to promote normality and minimise interventions, but on the other hand the dominance of risk management culture promotes a bio-medical model of care and defensive practise, contributing to increased interventions.

Davies et al (2000) offer an insight into organisation's culture by categorising organisational cultures as integrated, differentiated or fragmented. Integrated culture is defined as professionals working within it, having 'a wide consensus on the basic beliefs and appropriateness of behaviours within the organisation'. In an organization with integrated culture there is more likelihood of common goals, joint decision-making and sharing of philosophies underpinning care between the midwives and obstetricians.

On the whole, NHS organisations are more likely to fit a 'differentiated' cultural model because of a number of diverse groups of professionals and non-professionals with different value systems, views and norms all working together. In a fragmented culture the differences between staff groups are more marked than the commonalities between the various groups. It displays characteristics of 'shifting alliances and allegiances, considerable uncertainty and ambiguity, and unpredictability'. Davies et al (2000) conclude that all three types of cultures are prevalent in most NHS organisations to a greater or a lesser degree.

The Confidential Enquiries into Maternal Deaths and Child Health (CEMACH, 2007) recommends that partnership working between different professional groups, promotion of inter-professional learning and joint working between the professional organisations will contribute to understanding each other's roles and value systems. Professionals need to work together to promote integrated culture, which in turn offers scope to influence the outcomes of care delivery and improvement in staff morale and confidence.

The Healthcare Commission's review (HCC, 2005) of maternity units highlights lack of communication between professionals and failure to consider individual women's needs, resulting in sub-optimum care. They recognise the midwife as a key player and often is the only professional with whom women can build trusting relationship. Kirkham (2006) reports that while midwives are committed to building trusting relationships (and that this is the aspect of their job that they most enjoy), it is this very aspect that is compromised during the rationalisation of services. It is inevitable that during the rationalisation process midwifery posts are lost leading to a reduction in the number of midwives, yet their workload remains unchanged.

Hunter (2004) adds a further dimension to this debate. She asserts 'conflicting ideologies' operate between hospital and community midwifery practice:

> *'Hospital midwifery was dominated by meeting service needs, via a universalistic and medicalised approach to care; the ideology was, by necessity, "with institution". Community-based midwifery was more able to support an individualised, natural model of childbirth reflecting a "with woman" ideology'.*
>
> Hunter 2004: 270

Bosanquet (2005) argues that very large units, especially those with 8000 plus births per year, become unmanageable where monitoring of care and staffing become an onerous and complex process, further exacerbating their already stretched capability and capacity, with serious consequences to the safety of mothers and babies. Whilst the policy initiatives are ambitious in putting the women at the centre of care delivery, there is a widespread concern by the public and midwives over closures of birth centres and mergers of maternity units.

Management *versus* Professionals

The introduction of general management in the 1980s and internal market forces in the 1990s within the NHS have skewed the balance of power towards managerialism. The splitting of provider and purchaser functions in health services have increased management accountability and reinforced business values to a service industry (DH, 1997). The target culture has further legitimised the authority and dominance of managerialism. Managers have not only taken a dominant role in the contractual and human resource functions, but are also increasingly influencing the priorities and the organisation of clinical care.

The potential for conflict between managers and professionals arises from the different value system each holds. Drife and Jonstone (1995) argue that the managers have a vested interest in the survival of the whole organisation and its functions as opposed to the professionals whose primary responsibility is to deliver safe care, and expect the appropriate resources to ensure that. They also assert that the NHS is a community of managers, diverse professionals and support staff, each group having its own identity and culture. Each group makes demands on resources with its own priorities, thus leading to a tension between the professionals and the managers. Drife and Johnston (1995) conclude that the dominant management subculture is often perceived as a barrier to the clinicians' autonomy and freedom to practise.

Managers in the NHS have a responsibility for getting the work done that fulfils the obligations of providing a service that fits the tenets of the *Modern and Dependable NHS* (DH, 1997) and are accountable to the government for delivering the policy agenda. Managers are not only struggling to survive the impact of financial restraints, but also to meet the expectations of users and deliver the policy imperatives. For example, there has been pressure on the managers in maternity services to deliver choice agenda, provide one-to-one care model in labour, reduce interventions and at the same time introduce government targets of antenatal screening, accommodate reduction in junior doctors hours, and facilitate the development of new roles and skill mix.

Midwives are often deployed to undertake roles for which they are not always prepared to meet the service demands. Midwives' working environment is stressful in that sometimes basic equipment has to be shared between rooms. Midwives often feel overstretched, and are often required to work extra shifts to provide a safe level of service, and feel restricted in exercising the full scope of their role (Ball, 2002). This has the potential to leave a negative effect on student midwives' learning experiences.

Bosanquet et al (2005) argue that clinicians are increasingly having to take on additional workload generated through the clinical governance stream, for example risk management protocols, audit of care delivery, implementation of NICE guidelines, and to comply with numerous policy directives, thus further reducing the time allocated to clinical activity. Heavy reliance on protocols, guidelines and evidence-based care is seen by midwives as promoting a bio-medical model, resulting in midwives feeling devalued and being compromised in exercising their autonomy and intuitive clinical judgement. Midwives undertaking roles that do not reflect the full scope and activities of a midwife feel alienated from midwifery practice and aspects of their work that they enjoy

Increasing numbers of midwifery managers appear to have responsibilities without any authority. Their voice is often represented through the nursing hierarchy. The gap between the needs of clinical midwives and managers' responsibility to balance the policy imperatives and financial targets inevitably becomes wider, exacerbating the conflict and tension between the two groups.

Midwifery Leadership

Midwifery leadership has become increasingly important in a culture where the contradictions of rationalisation of services versus choices in models of care, budget deficits versus evidence-based quality care, reduction in skilled midwives, yet meeting the expectations of public are a daily reality for midwifery managers. During maternity services reconfiguration and closures, midwifery voice is often represented by the directors of nursing, thus limiting opportunity for midwifery leaders to inform and influence the decision-makers. Hence, it is not surprising that leadership in midwifery is underdeveloped (Shribman, 2007).

Gould (2005) argues that whilst midwives take refuge in 'passivity and fantasies to avoid unpleasant decisions', dominant professions continue to exert their values on midwifery. She asserts midwives 'need to wrestle with their inner need to conform and please others' and become politically engaged.

Consultant midwife posts were created to give a new career framework and provide a strong focus for clinical leadership (NHS, 1999) and to strengthen links between education, practice and research. Consultant midwives in the UK have taken on the challenge of clinical leadership by investing a considerable energy in promoting midwifery skills to support the physiological processes of pregnancy, labour and birth. However, the focus on clinical leadership has been distracted by competing priorities and service development initiatives. Consultant midwives have found themselves in a variety of roles, for example addressing social and health inequalities (Barber, 2002). Whilst addressing social and health inequalities is integral to the midwife's role and supporting vulnerable women is vital work, strong clinical midwifery leadership is needed in the clinical environment to strengthen midwifery skills, to promote normality, and contribute to the reduction of interventions.

Recently, dissent has been expressed within the profession and by the NHS trusts against those consultant midwives who focus their attention on supporting normal midwifery and strengthening practice. The common belief being that the labour ward coordinators are better placed to promote normality and midwifery skills. Consultant midwives are isolated in their endeavours as the numbers are still small (55 consultant midwives to date) and a number of posts have been lost through redundancies (personal communication). For midwifery to participate effectively in diversity of provision of care, reduction in interventions, one-to-one care in labour and the choice agenda, it is imperative that the number of consultant midwife posts need to be increased and be given legitimacy to challenge the current dominance of biomedical model in pregnancy and birth.

On an optimistic note Warwick (1996) suggests an 'effective voice depends on an ability to be heard...it is clear that purchasers and members of trust executives realise the value of listening to the experts'. However this means midwives taking responsibility and preparing a case for developing a service that meets the needs of local women.

Staffing of Maternity Services

The impact of skill mix, budget deficits, the demographic-time bomb, workforce strategy and changing patterns of work organisation, have influenced overall staffing in maternity services.

Evidence suggests that there is a reduction in the numbers of practising midwives (NMC, 2005; RCM, 2007). The reasons for the reduction are threefold; firstly there is a reduction (10-15%) in the number of places commissioned for midwifery education programmes, with serious consequences for the future. Secondly there is reduction in midwifery staffing establishments through freezing of senior midwifery posts and lack of midwifery posts for newly qualified midwives (RCM, 2007). Thirdly almost 30% of midwives are approaching retirement age and are most likely to leave due to the increasing stress and dissatifaction at work.

However, it has been argued that in order to meet the service needs the reduction in midwife numbers is compensated by promoting skill mix. The changes in workforce development range from developing new roles, for example assistant practitioner, to blurring the boundaries of existing roles. There is pressure on the providers of care to harness skill mix to release midwives' time and for them to take on complex and expanded roles. An RCM survey of heads of midwifery services confirmed that there is a trend towards reduction in the midwifery staffing establishments (RCM, 2006), and that increasing numbers of new roles are being developed. It also highlighted that midwives are experiencing fragmentation and substitution of their roles.

Increasing emphasis on role development and blurring of role boundaries is exacerbating student midwives' clinical experience, supervision and confidence and competence in supporting women during childbirth because the roles normally undertaken by student midwives are being delegated to support workers. Sandall et al (2007) highlight that maternity support workers are being trained to take on a range of clinical activities in some NHS trusts, for example newborn screening tests, post-Caesarean section observations, and post-natal visits in the community. This contributes to not only the fragmentation of care, but also to the substitution of roles. The move towards a health service dominated by care assistant roles may be a viable economic option, but its long-term impact on quality of care, research, innovation, evidence in health care, and existing professional roles has the potential to undermine clinical governance agenda and could have a detrimental effect on the health outcomes of mothers and babies. The impact of skill mix needs a robust evaluation to inform future workforce strategies.

Modernising Careers

A blue-print for *Modernising Nursing Careers* supported by the health departments of all four countries (DHSSPS, Scottish Executive, Welsh Assembly Government and DH, 2006) sets the direction for the future of nursing. Its emphasis on 'flexibility, balance between generalists and specialists and a career structure built around patient care pathways' suggests radical changes not only in the professional education programmes but also in service delivery. *Modernising Nursing Careers* aims to 'shatter the old demarcations which have held back staff and slowed down care' and ensure that the professionals' expertise is used more effectively. It envisages development of a flexible workforce with transferable skills and the breaking down of the traditional professional boundaries and tribalism.

Although *Modernising Nursing Careers* is in its embryonic stage, it is in the interests of midwives to analyse the impact of a career structure with increased number of care assistants and a flexible principle-based curriculum around patient pathway with a strong academic foundation and interdisciplinary learning. This will have implications not only on the future role of the midwife but also on the number of midwifery posts and the future of midwifery education. It will create a maternity service in which the majority of direct care may be provided by the MSWs whilst midwives with expertise are engaged in coordinating services and making strategic decisions.

The Modernising of professional careers is a commendable objective to develop a workforce that is adaptable and can meet the needs of women in the 21st century, but the resulting impact of eroding professional identity and the blurring of role boundaries may risk fracturing existing lines of responsibility and accountability.

Conflicts Experienced within the Midwifery Profession

The workforce modernisation in the NHS is impacting on the status, morale and identity of all healthcare professionals, and midwives are no exception. A culture of 'self-preservation' and 'self-serving community' of practitioners is emerging whereby the professionals are becoming disenfranchised and no longer feel able to take ownership of their professional practice (Ball et al, 2002), or support their peers or work in collaboration with other teams.

Professionalism or de-professionalism

Midwifery has secured its status as a profession through educational provision at diploma (Diploma Level will no longer be available from September 2008 [NMC, 2007]) and degree levels in higher education institutions and through its statutory regulatory framework. The midwife's role is grounded in statute with rules and code of practice (NMC, 2004) yet the meaning that midwives attribute to their work remains largely unexplored.

Fox (1980) suggests that the meaning of work is socially and culturally determined. He introduces two concepts to the meaning of work. The first concept considers that work is instrumental to earning wages, with the pursuit to accumulate wealth becoming a central focus. Midwives' in this category would be those who are happy to relinquish their clinical roles and responsibility. Although midwives in this particular group enjoy their work, they do not aspire to take on the challenges of service development or participating in alternative models of care. Their work is based on custom and practice model of how it is always done. The second concept considers work as an opportunity to self-actualisation, a source of satisfaction, work becoming a passion and integral to individual's value and belief system. Midwives in this group aspire to developing new midwifery knowledge and seek to strengthen midwifery practice

The dissonance between those whose work is instrumental to wages and those who see it as a means to status, personal identity and contribution to greater good becomes evident in the position each group occupies in the professional hierarchy. For example, those in the self-actualisation group gain promotion and their work becomes acknowledged faster than the midwives in the work as instrumental to wages group. Midwives who see their work as instrumental to wages limit the scope of their role, whereas those who see it as a means for stretching their potential push the boundaries and become champions for professional status, identity, and seek to advance the profession. It is inevitable that the two concepts embedded within the meaning of work creates a potential for conflict between the two groups due to different value systems.

Whilst the contractual agreements of wages, family friendly policies and flexible working are welcome, these could be construed as attributing to 'feminisation' of midwives' work. Hyman (1975) highlights a class and gender struggle with an imbalance of power between employees and employers. He suggests that employees can be manipulated and could be socialised into accepting policies introduced by those in power as a good thing. Hyman (1975) asserts employee needs and demands need to be considered within the wider economic and political context of society.

As health professionals' status, remuneration and position improve, the demand to fund highly skilled professionals, when the majority of the users require fundamental care, is being questioned (Shribman, 2007). Are initiatives of flexible working patterns, family friendly policies and organisation of midwives' work being introduced to fracture midwives' pivotal position in the maternity services? Also, the increasing costs of wages is challenging the politicians and the midwives need to question whether their expert knowledge and demand for appropriate remuneration is driving them out of service delivery market by being too expensive. Also, are the academic professional education programmes a requisite to all care delivery?

As the drive for skill mix gathers momentum, the identity of midwifery and other professions become proletarianised, their roles are expanded, deconstructed and they appear to increasingly take on the characteristics of salaried servants. Their status could be perceived to be relegated to a semi-profession or an occupation, the difference being subtle but nevertheless there.

The role of midwives and their professional identity is being continually shaped by external factors influencing the provision of maternity services. An increasing numbers of healthcare assistants are progressed through the knowledge and skills framework and are socialised into new ways of working employee functionality. This also contributes to a devaluing of professionals and therefore a degree of deprofessionalisation becomes inevitable.

The state control through regulation and the requirement of indemnity insurance for independent midwives is reinforcing the fit-for-purpose agenda. The professional values of autonomy and relationship with client are being eroded by national standards, patient care pathways and payment by results at the cost of professional freedom to practise.

Hierarchy Within the Profession

Midwifery is unique in that accountability at senior level appears to be shared. For example, typically a head of midwifery services does not often have a voice at the Trust Board level but she is represented by a Director of Nursing Services. Consultant midwives, although initially appointed to lead clinical practice, appear to focus more on service development, tackling health inequalities and are accountable to heads of midwifery services in some NHS Trusts. Finally the Local Supervising Authority Midwifery Officers are involved at strategic decision-making levels and yet their influence at local level seems patchy (Health Care Commission, 2005; Baron, 2007).

The remuneration of specialist roles through job evaluation profile is graded at a higher level within the *Agenda for Change* pay band, thus creating a division and tension between midwives striving to promote normality and using core/essential midwifery skills to strengthen midwifery practice.

Whilst career opportunities are welcome, it risks alienating midwives supporting the majority of women by working in mainstream settings of hospital and community and developing a discontinuity in the profession's identity, values and beliefs and creating a new hierarchy within the profession.

Tensions in Midwifery Education

The majority of healthcare professionals' education is embedded in professional, clinical and academic components and is delivered in higher education institutions at undergraduate level. Midwifery attracts qualified nurses to undertake a shortened pre-registration midwifery education programme at degree levels.

Anecdotal evidence suggests that a 78-week programme is too expensive to fund, and a number of providers are no longer able to recruit sufficient numbers to the shortened programme, hence the future of shortened midwifery education programme for registered nurses appears threatened. Other concerns include the programme being too short for student midwives to gain appropriate knowledge and skills, yet they bring a vast knowledge and skills of caring for high risk women and understanding of pathological changes in complicated pregnancies.

Shared/interprofessional learning programmes are being advocated as there is a strong belief that there are similarities in the majority of the content of healthcare professionals' programmes, and duplication in teaching these to different groups could be avoided by promoting shared learning (Frazer, 2002). Interprofessional education also fosters a better understanding of each other's roles and relationship between professionals.

The RCM Student Midwives Hardship survey (2004) found that two thirds of the student midwives entering the profession are already graduates. Should the profession consider developing a fast-track programme — which the medical profession has already addressed?

Finally, the social profile of midwifery students is changing; it ranges from experienced mature students, to parents with dependents, to school leavers, each group with different needs. An RCM survey (RCM, 2004) found that the average age of midwifery student is 29 years and that midwifery is their second career choice. They enter midwifery with expectations, pre-existing commitments and responsibilities. Student midwives experience contradictions and challenges with financial hardship, clinical placements and domestic commitments. On entry to the programme midwifery students are challenged with the expectation of being able to juggle academic, clinical and personal commitments all at the same time. Should midwifery education offer flexibility in the programme structure and develop a curriculum for part-time students to make the programme more widely accessible to this group of student midwives?

The nature and settings for clinical activity are constantly changing thus impacting on opportunities for student midwives to gain appropriate experience and acquire clinical skills. Clinical experience is further compromised for some student midwives due to the increasing number of maternity support workers and a lack of role models.

The reconfiguration of maternity services and other NHS reforms impact on the traditional systems and structures of clinical experiences. Recognition and reform of the hidden curriculum is required to identify the impact of NHS reforms on student midwives' clinical experience, and action needs to be taken to achieve the fundamental changes in the culture of clinical environment to enhance the learning experiences of all students (Lempp and Seale, 2004).

Opportunities for Midwives

Engaging with Partners

As the ideology of care provision changes from unilateral setting to plurality of providers, it offers midwives the opportunity to practise not only in different settings but also work in partnership with different providers. Now is the time for midwives to engage and build alliances and allegiances with general practitioners and independent sectors.

Midwives need to develop strategies to strengthen their skills and knowledge to lead midwifery services in all settings and to work in partnership with all providers of maternity services. There is a scope for building on existing alliances and working with partners to promote holistic models of care. The profession needs to strengthens its practice base, and become part of a pluralist system, with women, medical staff, midwives and other team players as stakeholders; there is a scope for developing shared multi-professional standards for supporting all learners with equal access to appropriate clinical experience.

Using Policy Initiatives as Levers for Change

A midwife's role is grounded in statute; there is an established supervision network and a statutory standard to ensure they remain fit for practise (NMC, 2004). The NHS reforms, especially the policies on maternity services, can be viewed as an opportunity for midwives to not only strengthen their status and position in the modern NHS, but perhaps to contribute to shaping and forming sustainable structures that will embed the principles of women-centred maternity care and make choice agenda a reality (DH and DfES, 2004). Midwives are ideally placed to embed the vision and standards outlined in the National Service Frameworks.

Midwives have an opportunity to embed the policy imperatives of choice, service level agreements and inequalities in health targets to support women from vulnerable backgrounds and improve health care outcomes for these women. They are in a pivotal position to establish partnership working between different agencies, for example social services, prison services strategic health authorities and voluntary organizations and access funding from non traditional sources.

Midwifery Roles

Over the last decade midwives have become engaged in a range of specialist roles; some of these have been advocated nationally and others have emerged as part of service development initiatives at local level. A number of these roles are at strategic level, giving midwives an opportunity to influence maternity services' provision at strategic level — for example the consultant midwives in some areas are working in partnership with social services and local authorities to provide continuity of care based on total needs of women and their families through life cycle. Midwives have embraced the Sure Start scheme (Sure Start Unit, 2005) and are integrating public health dimensions of their roles to support women and their families They are working with the commissioners and other stakeholders — including users — to look at the whole system approach to review the current provision of maternity services. It is anticipated that midwives at leadership level will also make substantial contributions to the maternity services review announced by the Health Care Commission and King's Fund in 2007.

Midwives, in their roles as antenatal screening coordinators, are the key professionals taking the responsibility for translating, implementing and evaluating the antenatal national screening programme at local level. They have been at the forefront of developing guidelines and training for midwives on information giving, choices and accessing counseling services for women. They are in a unique position to raise the profile of midwifery.

Consultant midwives have been appointed to provide clinical leadership, and this legitimises their role in supporting midwives to gain confidence and competence in midwifery skills and champion the promotion of normality and reduction in interventions. The profession needs to support the consultant midwives and resist any pressure from the employers to make these senior posts redundant. Their role is integral to delivering the National Service Framework standards of meeting the needs of socially excluded women and meeting the maternity services targets of improving breastfeeding rates, reduction in teenage pregnancies and the choice agenda.

Local Supervising Authority Midwifery Officers have overall responsibility of supervision of practice. By working with Heads of Midwifery services, consultant midwives and Lead midwives for education they can influence the direction of maternity services that best serves the women and their families.

Leadership

There is an urgent need in midwifery to develop and provide opportunities for leadership at all levels. Although there are numerous leadership initiatives supported by health departments of all four countries, these appear to be a low priority at local level. Midwifery education has a vital role in supporting and developing continuing professional development for midwifery managers at local level.

It is imperative that midwifery managers become committed to strengthening clinical leadership and raising the profile of midwifery care models within the mainstream maternity services. Midwifery leaders need to evaluate the impact of skill mix, PRB schemes, and collect evidence to influence decision makers. Does the skill mix agenda effectively address the reduction in establishment numbers of midwives and the resulting expert-skill shortage?

Kirkham (2006) highlights the fundamental priority for a midwifery manager is to align the professional aspirations of midwives with the aspirations of the women within the restrictions of the service demands.

Organisational Level

Midwives continue to challenge the positioning of maternity services in acute sector for all women. They have overcome the barriers of the traditional model of maternity services to develop birth centres and midwife led units to not only embrace choice agenda but also to promote normality and holistic model of care (RCM, 2000). However, midwives need to consider seriously the economic viability of birth centres and midwife-led care. The Albany Group Practice (Sandall, 2001) developed by midwives, now subcontracted by acute sector, is unique and sustainable, it is designed around women's needs and it integrates the normality agenda with mainstream maternity services. Midwives working in the 'Practice' provide continuity of care to women in their own surroundings, thus building trusting relationships, and influencing women's lifestyles towards a healthy start for their unborn babies.

Independent midwives are paid by women who use their services. Many of the independent midwives opted out of the NHS to give the kind of care that is being advocated by the maternity service frameworks. Independent midwives believe they have the experience, knowledge and skills to provide holistic woman-centred care and are currently negotiating with the NHS providers to be subcontracted in order to offer an alternative care model to those women who wish to use it.

Further opportunities are available for midwives to engage in social enterprise models, as the government pursues its goal of encouraging pluralist providers of care. Midwives can become independent providers of care or become equal partners in existing primary care centres and GP practices.

Midwives have taken the opportunity to address inequalities and other priorities to improve outcomes for women and their families. Midwives have negotiated specialist roles to develop services and support the most vulnerable in our society, for example coordinator roles have emerged for pregnant teenagers, asylum seekers, substance abusers, pregnant women in prisons, abuse from violence and a number of others. However, these roles need to be integrated into mainstream maternity services and used to raise the profile of midwifery.

Midwives in leadership roles at general manager levels are ideally placed to work in collaboration with consultant midwives, midwifery educationalists and Local Supervising Authority Midwifery Officers to influence decisions at the Trust Board levels and strategy levels to make maternity services a priority with long-term benefits to the future citizens of UK.

Despite the reduction in the number of midwives, midwives continue to spend substantial proportion of their time on non-clinical activities. Can midwives afford to continue undertaking non-midwifery duties and delegating essential/core midwifery skills to non-midwives?

Can midwives continue to attribute meaning of their work as being instrumental to wages and retain the existing agenda for change pay bands, or should we be moving more towards 'meaning of work' as being instrumental to higher goals of being more about self-actualisation and that of a professional?

As the settings for providing maternity services expand, midwives may benefit by taking a professional approach and evaluating the value and meaning of their work. In order to sustain their position and status with the diverse providers of maternity services midwives may need to consider making a shift from an employee status to a professional clinician and to increasingly work in partnership with women, other professionals and consumer groups.

Activity 10

1. Give two examples of the conflicts that you have experienced as a student midwife.

2. In your opinion how can some contradictions experienced by midwives in practice be resolved?

References

Anderson T (2007) Is this end of independent midwifery? *The Practising Midwife* **10**(2): 4-5

Ball J (1996) *Birth-rate Plus: a Framework for Workforce Planning and Decision Making for the Maternity services*. Books for Midwives, Cheshire

Ball L, Curtis P, Kirkham M (2002) *Why do Midwives Leave?* RCM, London

Barber T (2002) Consultant midwives: cameos from clinical practice. *RCM MIDWIVES Journal* **5**(5): 166-169

Baron J (2007) The conservative view. *RCM MIDWIVES Journal* **10**(3): 110

Barrell M (2004) Our destiny in our hands. *The Practising Midwife* **7**(5): 4-5

Bosanquet N, Ferry J, Lees C, Thornton J (2005) Maternity services in the NHS. Reform, London

Confidential Enquiries into Maternal Deaths and Child Health (2007) *Saving Mother's lives: Reviewing maternal deaths to make motherhood safer 2003-2005*. CEMACH, London

Healthcare Commission (2005) *State of Healthcare 2005 [annual report]*. Healthcare Commission, London

Crisp N (2005) *Commissioning a PatientlLed NHS*. Department of Health, London

Davies HT, Nutley S, Mannion R (2000) Organisational culture and quality of health care. *Quality in Health Care* **9**: 111-119

DH/NHS (1999) *Making a Difference: strengthening the nursing, midwifery and health visiting contribution to health and healthcare*. DoH, London

DH (2000) *NHS Plan: A Plan for Investment — A Plan for Reform*. DH, London

DH (2000) *A Health Service of all the Talents Developing the NHS. Workforce consultation document on the review of workforce planning*. DH, London

DH (2001) *Tackling Health Inequalities Consultation on a Plan for Delivery*. DH, London

DH (2004a) *The NHS Knowledge and Skills Framework (NHS KSF) and the Development Review Process*. DH, London

DH (2004b) *NHS Job Evaluation Handbook*. 2nd ed. DH, London

DH (2004c) *National Service Framework for Children, Young People and Maternity services — Maternity Services*. DH, and DfES, London

DfES (2004d) *National Service Framework for Children, Young People and Maternity Services. Maternity services*. DH and DfES, London.

DH (2006a) *Our Health, Our Care, and Our Say: A new direction for community services. Cmnd 6737*. TSO, Norwich

DH (2006b) *Modernising Bursary Scheme*. DH, London

DH (2006c) Modernising Nursing Careers — Setting the Direction. DH, London

DH (2007) *The New NHS: Modern and Dependable*. DH, London

DH (2007) *Options for the Future of Payment by Results: 2008/2009 to 2010/2011*. DH, London

Drife J, Johnston I (1995) Management for Doctors: Handling the conflicting cultures in the NHS. *BMJ* **310**: 1054-1056

Fox A (1980) The meaning of work. In: Esland G, Salaman G, eds. *The Politics of Work and Occupations*. Open University Press, Milton Keynes

Fraser DM (2000) Action Research to improve the pre-registration midwifery curriculum Part 2: case study evaluation in seven sites in England. *Midwifery* **16**(4): 277-286

Gould D (2005) It is time for our leaders to emerge. *British Journal of Midwifery* **13**(1): 11

Health Care Commission (2007) *Maternity Services Review*. Healthcare Commission, London

Hunter B (2004) Conflicting ideologies as a source of emotion work in midwifery. *Midwifery* **20**(3): 261-72

Hyman R (1975) *Industrial Relations: Marxist Introduction*. Macmillan, London

Kendall L, Lissauer R (2003) *The Future Healthcare Worker*. The Institute of Public Policy and Research, London

Kings Fund (2007) *Enquiry into Maternity Services*. Kings Fund, London

Kirkham M (1999) The culture of midwifery in the National Health Service in England. *Journal of Advanced Nursing* **30**(3): 732-739

Kirkham M, Morgan RK, Davies C (2006) *Why Do Midwives Stay?* RCM, London

Kotter JP (19990) *What Leaders Really Do*. Harvard Business Review **May/June**: 103-111

Lewis R, Hunt P, Carson D (2006) *Social Enterprise and Community — Based Care. Is there a future for mutually owned organisations in community and primary care?* Kings Fund, London

Manero E (2003) *Changes and Closures of Maternity Services in England. Making the Voice of Users Hear: Making the Voice of Users Hear*. The National Childbirth Trust, London

National Assembly for Wales (2001) *Improving Health in Wales: A plan for NHS and its partners.* NHS Wales, Cardiff

National Health Service Employers (2005) *Agenda for Change: NHS Terms and conditions of Service Handbook.* DH, London

National Health Service Quality Improvement Scotland (2005) *Clinical Standards – Maternity Services.* NHS Quality Improvement Scotland, Edinburgh

NMC (2004a) *Standards of Proficiency for Pre–registration Midwifery Education.* NMC, London

NMC (2004b) *Guidance on Provision of Midwifery Care and Delegation of Midwifery Care.* NMC Circular 01/2004. NMC, London

NMC (2005) *Statistical Analysis of the Register from 1st April 2004 to 31st March 2005.* NMC, London

NMC (2006) *Standards to Support Learning and Assessment in Practice.* NMC, London

RCM (2000) *Vision 2000.* RCM, London

RCM (2004) Student Hardship Survey. *RCM MIDWIVES Journal* **October 2004:** Mid-month Supplement

RCM (2007) RCM evidence to the pay review body. *RCM MIDWIVES Journal* **10**(1): 6

Sandall J, Davies J, Warwick C (2001) *Evaluation of the Albany Midwifery Practice: Final Report.* King's College, London

Sandall J.(2007) Maternity support workers roles – personal communication

National Health Service in Scotland (2001) *Our National Health: A plan for action: A plan for Change.* Stationery Office, Edinburgh

Shen J, Cox A, McBride A (2004) Factors influencing turnover and retention of midwives and consultants: a literature review. *Health Services Management Research* **17**(4): 249-262

Shribman S (2007) *Making it Better for Mother and Baby: Clinical case for change.* DH, London

Sure Start Unit (2005) *A Sure Start Children's Centre for Every Community: Phase 2 planning and guidance (2006-2008).* Sure Start, London

Walsh D (2007) *Improving Maternity Services: Small is beautiful – lessons from a birth centre.* Radcliffe Publishing, Oxford

Welsh Assembly Government (2005) *National Service Framework for Children, Young People and Maternity Services in Wales.* Welsh Assembly Government, London

Warwick C (1996) Leadership in midwifery care. *British Journal of Midwifery* **4**(5): 229

CHAPTER 11

My Journey

Lorna Muirhead

I was delighted to be asked to write my personal journey recounting the experiences of 40 years of midwifery practice. As I put the pen to paper, not only the memories of changes and enormous strides in education and knowledge of childbirth have occurred flooded my thoughts. I also became aware of the incidents that have shaped my views and opinions.

I trained as a midwife in Birmingham in 1964, but spent most of my working life in Liverpool. My passion is the care received by women during labour. I spent 35 years doing just that, briefly leaving the clinical area for two years to become a 'sister tutor' (today that would be a midwifery lecturer). In 1993 I was elected to Council of the Royal College of Midwives (RCM) and in 1997 became its President, a post I held for almost eight years.

This chapter aims to highlight the context in which midwives practised in the 1960s before the institutionalisation of childbirth in hospitals. It seeks to provide rational for increased medicalisation and inverventions and explores principles and value systems that continue to impact on the midwife's role and midwifery practice. The experiences I have encountered will strike a chord with not only with my contemporaries, but also with the student midwives pursuing undergrade studies in the first decade of the 21st century despite advances in technology, midwifery education and evidence based knowledge.

The Beginning

The bell rang and I and three other new pupil midwives (as they were then called), trying to master the art of palpation, left the ante-natal clinic and rushed to labour ward to witness our first delivery.

It was 1964, when childbirth was not viewed as the normal life-changing event which it is today, but as a frightening painful experience which women had to endure in order to become mothers; a time when ante-natal education was almost non-existent and women came to childbirth hardly knowing what to expect. Many were forced to deliver at home because there were not enough maternity beds for them to have their baby in hospital, which is what women then aspired to do. Hospital birth was becoming all the rage!

Labours were longer and were experienced without the support of husbands and family, who generally left the women at the labour ward door.

Women laboured with inadequate pain relief in 'Nightingale style' wards — with numerous beds and only a curtain separating them. There was minimal privacy or presence of supportive partners. Women supported each other and shared their experiences. The year 1964 predated epidural analgesia, so easily dismissed today, but not by midwives of my generation who knew the onerous and draining experience of sitting with women in agony experiencing prolonged or painful labour. When epidural analgesia was first used for such labours I was its most ardent supporter, and I remain so even now, although with some reservation.

Eliminating Risk

More women died in childbirth then than they do today. Between 1964 and 1966 a total of 954 maternal deaths were recorded (DHSS, 1986). The main complication which killed women was post-partum haemorrhage. The routine use of Syntometrine and the active management of the third stage of labour, which has largely eradicated this condition, certainly from vaginal delivery, was some way off.

The Triennial Confidential Enquiries into Maternal Deaths (DHSS, 1986) (the fore-runner of CEMACH) contained accounts of the deaths of women who had inhaled vomit at emergency Caesarean section and died of Mendelson's syndrome. As a result, women in labour were fed a liquid diet of soup, jelly and ice cream, and sucked glucose sweets. Perhaps when reviewing whether or not women should be fed in labour today, the reasons why they were ever not fed should be borne in mind.

Prematurity was considered to be anything under 36 weeks gestation. Special Care baby units did not exist, although there were a few premature baby units. The year 1964 predated the contraceptive pill and the Abortion Act, and there were many unplanned pregnancies for married and unmarried women alike. It was a huge social disgrace to be pregnant out of wedlock, so much so that girls finding themselves in this situation used to go 'on holiday' to another town where they delivered their child, often having it adopted, and then conveniently arrived back home 'from holiday'.

It will be difficult for today's midwife to contemplate childbirth or the practice of midwifery within this context; just as in 40 years time it will be difficult for the midwives of the day to contemplate the practice you do now. Professional life moves on, and goalposts and expectations constantly move.

The preoccupation of the professionals caring for pregnant women when I trained was to eliminate risk from childbirth. As professionals it was mandatory that we should do so, and women expected no less from us. The attempt to eliminate risk led to the use of routine procedures for all women, which in turn meant that some women could be said to have been over-monitored and over-treated, but this blanket approach to care has undoubtedly played a significant part in making birth in the UK as safe as it is today.

However, it could be said, that in making it so, there is a danger of our becoming victims of our own success, resulting in some of those procedures which make birth safe now being abandoned. This is very much like the current thinking on vaccinating all children against measles. No-one believes that all children who contract measles will be damaged or die, but some will, and since it is impossible to accurately predict those children who will, vaccination of all children is advised. If many children were dying in this country during an outbreak of measles, there would be little reluctance in modern parents about having children vaccinated. But this is not happening, and parents can be forgiven for thinking that because they never hear of such tragedy they need not accept the very minimal risk associated with measles vaccination. Likewise, birth is so successful and safe in the UK that we are letting down our guard, with the risk of becoming too complacent and missing the danger signals.

I accept the idea of low-risk and high-risk pregnancy, but it is worth reminding ourselves that there is no such thing as a no-risk pregnancy, which makes me feel justified with meticulous monitoring and appropriate intervention of those in my care. Successful though birth is at the beginning of the twenty-first century, success cannot be guaranteed prospectively. It can only be classified as successful, retrospectively.

My First Experience of a Delivery

As I approached the labour ward I felt mounting apprehension and anxiety, but at the same time excitement at the prospect of witnessing my first delivery. However the awful screams heard in the corridor meant that anxiety was my uppermost emotion. I had rarely heard such distress. As a nurse I had witnessed people badly injured and desperately needing help sounding so agonised, but this was a woman at the height of labour about to deliver her child. We, the three new pupils, stood at the foot of the bed, silent, frightened and fearful for the woman. She pushed, screamed and shouted, and then a non-breathing blue head suddenly appeared at the vulva.

There was a temporary silence. '*Why doesn't someone do something?*', I thought. '*The baby is surely dead*', I thought, since hitherto anything I had seen that colour and not breathing had been dead. The midwife in charge however was calm, tranquil and very unworried: she had a wonderful face. Another mighty scream from the woman and it was all over. Miraculously the child shuddered into life. I stood transfixed. I had just witnessed the most awesome, terrifying, painful experience I could imagine — but the mother, child in her arms, was now smiling. I left the room totally confused, found the nearest lavatory, and I wept.

Eventually my time came to work on labour ward and during the following six months I would witness, and become involved in, the most exciting, unpredictable, totally absorbing, painful process, called labour. I would help 84 women to deliver their babies and my lifelong passion for the care of labouring women would become established.

The labours which, in common with all midwives, I like best, are those which proceed normally and allow me to practise 'autonomously'. However, I strongly believe that midwives are there for all pregnant women, and my clinical practice over many years has embraced natural, normal, complicated, and alas, fatal childbirth. The latter two of those requiring me to move into a different gear of midwifery and become an equal partner of a multidisciplinary team, working towards the optimum outcome for mother and child. Dear to me though 'autonomous' midwifery is, it is secondary to doing what is necessary to secure the best outcome.

Experiences as a Student Midwife

And so, the first six months training was coming to an end. Perhaps I should tell you a bit about it. Midwifery was taught by 'Sister Tutors' within maternity hospitals. Every three months each training hospital took their required number of new pupils, who were not only guaranteed a job at the end of training, but indeed were expected, as new midwives, to work in their training hospital to give back some service.

Midwifery training was divided into Part I which covered all the theory of midwifery, and Part II, which largely involved public health and complicated childbirth. Part I was largely spent in hospital setting and Part II was on 'the district, which is now referred to as in 'the community'.

I bought a very old bicycle from a pupil midwife just returning from the district, was measured for my brown mackintosh and hat and collected my midwife's bag before cycling to the midwives' house in the middle of a council housing estate in Birmingham. The plaque on the door read 'Midwives' House'. Inside lived two district midwives, and every three months two new pupil midwives came to live and work with them. It was like a monastic life, totally immersed in midwifery.

What a wonderful experience I had with Janet Webb and Doris Eaves! They lived and worked amongst those they attended and were regarded as pillars of the community. Dressed in their green uniform they looked like the woman on the Quaker Oats packet; and yes, both drove Morris Minor cars. They knitted baby clothes, they ran ante-natal clinics, they did some 50 deliveries at home each year, and whilst I was with them I did 21. They were mistresses in the art of midwifery and taught me so much. I spoke at Miss Webb's funeral in 2003. This year (2006) Miss Eaves, now 92, still lives independently in Birmingham.

Daily I would be given my work, which was to attend ante-natal clinics, and to visit post-natal women (which we did for 10 days after delivery). Such visits included bed bathing the mother — few had bathrooms — bathing the child, making the bed, and checking temperature, pulse, respiration, lochia and the fundal height, and sometimes vacuum cleaning or doing some shopping for the family.

I particularly remember one birth I attended: a gravida four booked for home birth went into labour when I was in the Midwives' House alone. There was a knock at the door. *'Can you come to my mother?'*, said a little boy, *'she's going to have her baby'*. This mother, in common with most, had no telephone. I cycled to her home carrying all the equipment I needed, and arrived at the house to hear sounds which, had I been a little more experienced, I would have recognised as a woman approaching the second stage of labour. I ran, breathless from my cycle-ride, up the stairs. Keen to do the right thing and get the procedures right, and frightened that I was on my own, I took out my razor to shave the vulva. (In 1964 it was not humanly possible to deliver without a shaved vulva.) One swift move of the razor and the head of the child appeared with the centre of its head shaved! Seeing a bonnet which was laid out neatly on the dressing table ready to be put on the baby when it was born I seized it and put it on the head still at the vulva. Was this the first child in history actually delivered wearing a hat? When Miss Webb arrived she complimented me on my putting on a bonnet because the room was a little cold. The mother smiled, and we kept our little secret.

The next three months taught me a lot. Women mainly delivered their babies usually in the back bedroom of their parent's house as few young couples had accommodation of their own. Houses usually had no bathrooms and no telephone. Midwives had to rely on the telephone box in the street to summon aid if necessary.

Home birth, as ever, was wonderful when all went well, but if there was foetal distress, post-partum haemorrhage, sudden eclampsia, or a baby not breathing, home birth was a nightmare. In such circumstances it was left to the husband to run to find a working telephone and ring the local hospital, who would send out the flying squad.

The Flying Squad

The flying squad consisted of an ambulance which was always available, which brought to the patient's house a team consisting of an obstetrician, an anaesthetist, a midwife and a medical student. With them they brought blood and the equipment necessary to deal with conditions like ante-partum haemorrhage, post-partum haemorrhage, retained placenta, delay in second stage, eclampsia, undiagnosed breech, or twins in the second stage. Some of these conditions were dealt with at home, but if needs be the patient's condition was stabilised before she was transferred to hospital.

Flying squads were very much the predecessors of today's paramedics. The maternity services long ago knew that to transfer a compromised, pregnant woman to hospital by ambulance could result in death, and so the idea of initiating treatment which would make the patient safe at the scene before taking them to hospital, was born.

Although the flying squad usually arrived within half an hour of being called, half an hour was a life-time with a woman having an eclamptic fit, a woman haemorrhaging, or a second twin lying transversely. Perhaps this is why I have reservations and cannot share the contemporary views about the merit of home birth, or birth in free-standing maternity units, for all women.

Qualified Midwife

So my time in Birmingham ended — I passed Part II and was now a midwife. I had no thought of going back to nursing. During my midwifery training I met and fell in love with a tall, dark, handsome Scot who was at university in Aberdeen. He was going to Liverpool University to do a PhD and so I looked in the midwifery journals for a vacant post in Liverpool and saw the advertisement for a staff nurse at Liverpool Maternity Hospital. I had never been to Liverpool, I had never heard the accent, and I knew little about the area.

I arrived at Lime Street Station and walked up the hill to the hospital. The Matron, Emily Carter, met me. She had the face of a Madonna and was a visionary midwife who ran a hospital with standards for women and midwifery which were the very best of the day. I did not know then just how lucky I was to be successful in getting a job.

Unlike the place where I trained, Liverpool Maternity Hospital was a teaching hospital, which meant that it was attached to a medical school and had the brightest and best doctors and midwives working at it. It was also much better staffed and had a much bigger budget.

I thought I had gone to work in paradise. Women laboured in single rooms in a state of the art labour ward. Their husbands were 'allowed' to stay but only for normal deliveries. Liverpool was well ahead when it came to preparing women for labour and motherhood, and it ran 'mothercraft' preparation classes.

For labour the hospital offered women the Liverpool cocktail (or 'coughdrop' as the locals called it). This was 100mg of pethidine, 10mg morphine, and

200mg of butobarbitone given together when the cervix was 2cm dilated. It was topped up hours later with another 100mg of pethidine if required, followed by Entonox given at the end of the first stage and into the second stage of labour. Women slept throughout labour and often almost through delivery. Many a woman was heard to ask sometime later *'Did I have my baby?'* So much for bonding — but at least they were spared unwanted agony!

It is often asked: *'Surely all the babies were born with low APGARS?'* I can assure you they were not. At that time, the mid 1960s, there was no resident paediatrician in most maternity hospitals, which meant that midwives had to deal with all the babies born. Believe me, if babies had been born compromised by the analgesia which their mothers were given in labour, the analgesia would have been modified! After delivery, women were served a tray of tea. I had never seen this. A hurried drink from a communal teapot had been the norm where I previously worked — but a tray of tea!

In the post-natal wards women rested for 10 days. Their babies lived in a nursery where they were looked after by midwives and nursery nurses, and only taken to the mother to be fed. Surprisingly enough to the modern midwife, mothers did manage to bond with them. Post-natal wards outside feeding time were tranquil places where women spent time getting over birth. Midwives had time to devote to assisting with breastfeeding and teaching mothers how to bath and generally look after their babies. Post-natal wards were not, as they are today, like Heathrow airport, full of women coming and going.

I was exposed to Liverpool humour almost on my first day as I asked a woman I was booking: *'Name; address; religion; next of kin?'* *'Oh'* said the woman, *'I don't have a next of kin'*. *'What about your husband?'* I asked. *'Oh! he doesn't have one either'*, replied the woman.

The next week on the labour ward, looking after a labouring woman, I said to her: *'Don't you think you ought to have something for your pain?"* She seemed in agony to me. She retorted: *'I don't know! You're the b*****
midwife!'* This response tells you something about the relationship between patient and professionals at that time. That woman expected me, a qualified midwife, to advise her and to tell her what I thought would be best for her. This today is called paternalism, but I see some merit in women asking midwives what they think is best for them individually and the midwife giving the women the benefit of her midwifery education, knowledge and experience. Why else are we a profession?

Post 1970s

The *Peel Report* of 1970 (DHSS, 1970), now much castigated by many midwives, recommended on the grounds of safety that all births should take place in hospital. Today's midwives are dismissive of this because his evidence was not 'research-based'. Can I remind the reader that most of what we did then and do now is not research based; indeed until relatively recently we had little formal research to guide us but we still had a very successful profession.

Important though it is, let us keep research in its place as only one of the disciplines which informs us about practice.

What we did have in 1970 were statistics, presented in the Triennial Confidential Enquiries into Maternal Deaths (DHSS, 1986), which catalogued where and why deaths and morbidity occurred. The report supported Peel's conclusions that many of the deaths reviewed could have been avoided if the woman had been in the right place with the right equipment and the right level of expertise to hand. I share Peel's view (DHSS1970).

Post 1970 most babies were born in hospital, and statistical evidence supports the view that maternal and perinatal deaths declined. All women were now booked under obstetricians, who consequently believed that they bore responsibility for all pregnancies. In the attempt to improve labour, especially prolonged labour which was a common problem, obstetricians rightly intervened in intra-partum care to rectify conditions like cervical dystocia and incoordinate uterine action, so rarely seen today that modern midwives will have to resort to midwifery history books to identify it.

However, soon interventions spilled over into normal labour, with doctors believing that they had a duty to do what they considered best for all women in both complicated and normal labour. Those of us in practice at the time were just too busy getting on with the job to notice this insidious intervention in normal labour or the erosion of our role.

This is not a comfortable conclusion for me to reach, since it was my generation which was responsible for it. But let us not demonize doctors. They were doing what they thought was best for women, and I deplore the current anti-doctor attitude which some display. A strong, confident profession like midwifery does not need to demonise other professions, especially our obstetric colleagues who have played a vital part in making childbirth as good and safe as it is today. Now, there's an unfashionable view! Midwives do not have the monopoly of altruism. We did not on our own make the experience of childbirth the comparatively wonderful experience which it is today in this part of the world.

For all the interventions of the 1970s and 1980s do not for one minute think that all was bad for women then. I have no misty eyed nostalgia for childbirth at the beginning of my career or during those later years. On balance having a baby in this country gets better all the time and will continue to get better provided today's midwives keep the best practice of yesterday and marry it with the best of today's. Do not be tempted to throw the baby out with the bath water. As a young midwife I could only see as far as I could see, because I was standing on the shoulders of the generation of midwives who went before me. Today's midwives can only see as far as they can because they are standing on the shoulders of my generation. When today's midwives believe that they have found a better way of looking after pregnant women, they must avoid the temptation of rubbishing the efforts of the midwives who went before them who, like them, were giving care which conformed to the philosophy and best practice of their day.

Changing Demands

Let me remind you about some of the advances for women in the 1970s and 1980s, since some balance needs to be given to the very negative attitudes which midwives have about that time when the contraceptive pill which gave women more control over their fertility, and the Abortion Act had been passed in 1967.

Single rooms were provided for women to labour in privacy. The vast majority of women wanted effective pain relief during labour, and attention was paid to improving what was on offer. A marvellous innovation called epidural analgesia was introduced into labour-ward practise and midwives of the day adapted their management of labour, especially the second stage, so that the forceps rate did not rise dramatically, as one is led to believe. In my view, it is often incorrect management of the second stage of labour which leads to forceps or ventouse delivery, not epidural analgesia *per se*.

The introduction of continuous foetal monitoring meant that because the well-being of the foetus could be clearly seen, relaxation of the time limits imposed on the second stage was possible, and this was greatly welcomed. The second stage of labour was known to be a time of increased risk for the foetus, and my generation were exposed to catastrophic and unexpected intra-partum stillbirths. We welcomed continuous foetal monitoring! Foetal scanning and choice about continuing the pregnancy in the case of abnormality became available.

Special Care Baby Units (SCBU) were being set up everywhere, which meant that babies born spontaneously premature had more chance of survival. It also meant that conditions in the mother, such as severe pre-eclampsia, requiring very early delivery, became less of a problem. It would be good for today's midwives to pause and think about how difficult it was to manage complicated labours without SCBU.

Organisations like the National Childbirth Trust (NCT) were born and set up classes in ante-natal education and preparation for birth. However the NCT cannot, and does not, take all the credit for this because many midwives ran the same type of preparation classes.

This meant that for the first time women came to pregnancy and birth with some idea of what to expect. What was not so desirable in this context was that women soon began to have very fixed ideas about what they 'wanted' from their childbirth experience, regardless of whether their actual childbirth performance could support this or not.

This led to some disquiet amongst midwives who, until that time, were used to being consulted by pregnant women who asked for advice and usually took it. This is now called paternalism and is deeply unfashionable. However, in my view it is desirable for professionals to believe that they should know more than even the most well informed 'consumer', and midwives know exactly what women want to achieve by the end of their pregnancy.

We talk today about individualised care, but all birth plans in my experience, include most of the same things, and are not individual at all. We know that women want things to be as normal and uncomplicated as possible. They want to take home a healthy child and be proud of their achievement. They also want to be satisfied with the care they received. We want those things too! But midwives also know that this sort of childbirth is not women's to demand, or in the midwives' gift. It would be worth taking a few minutes to think about that.

Post 1980s

By the late 1980s midwives could have been forgiven for believing that childbirth was very good in terms of women's and babies survival, but the price for this was the over-medicalisation of childbirth.

We were now at a time when fertility was largely under women's control, and when scans almost guaranteed the normality of the baby. There were major advances in the survival of neonates, and women experienced shorter labours and had choice about the method of pain relief. They laboured in private with the support of families. These advances had taken many years to achieve through the efforts of my generation of midwives. I do not accept a common view that everything which happened to women at that time was undesirable, or that women could not have been happy or fulfilled with their childbirth experience. But times change, and periodic review of the maternity services and midwives' practice is essential.

No one welcomed more than I did the recommendations of *Changing Childbirth* (DH, 1993) because it heralded the renaissance of autonomous midwifery in the care of low risk women. However I remain to be convinced that in order to achieve this birth should be removed from hospital into the home, or into free-standing birth units. I completely support total midwifery care for low risk women, but my preference would be for it to take place in hospital with all emergency facilities to hand. The success of low risk birth in hospital lies in midwives and obstetricians 'getting their act together' and having mutual respect for each other, as indeed they have done far more frequently than some would have us believe.

As a profession we should be concerned with equity of care. What removing birth to the home or birthing units has done is to provide a minority of women a place where a lot of attention has been paid to making a homely environment, and providing them with one-to-one midwifery support in labour. However, today the majority of women labour in hospital, where often less attention has been paid to the physical environment, and midwives frequently look after two or three women with varying risk factors at one time. Whilst congratulating midwives in birthing units and those involved in home births for the care they give, in my view, the fact that birth experience is generally so highly rated in those areas has much to do with environment and staffing ratios. If midwives worked in hospitals where similar attention was given to the physical environment, and where they were able to give one-to-one care to women with similar risk factors, I wonder what evaluations would be like. After all, one-to-one care is supposed to be available to all women. At the moment we are comparing apples and pears.

Changing Childbirth fails to address adequately the needs of a very significant number of women for whom birth is complicated, or the practice of midwives who attend them. The experience of birth for these women is often viewed as second-rate, as is the practice of the midwife who attends them.

It seems to me that we live in a time where 'good birth' and 'good midwifery' is thought to be practised at home or in birthing units, and anything else, especially birth in hospital, is 'bad birth', and 'not proper midwifery'. This is to be deeply regretted and does not serve mother or midwives well. I believe that midwives are there for all women, and although the practice I enjoyed most was that which I could do autonomously when everything remained normal, I had no problem at all in moving up a gear to practice midwifery within a multidisciplinary team, in the care of women experiencing difficulty. Many I know share this view.

Midwives have to guard against becoming too idealistic and too pure. As a profession we should make no apology about having a philosophy which supports non-intervention and normal birth, but we must beware that this philosophy does not become an ideology which results in our not intervening when it is necessary to do so. Having castigated obstetricians for intervening unnecessarily, midwives today must not be guilty of failing to intervene when it is essential. Herein lies the wisdom of practice.

Natural versus Normal childbirth

It seems to be increasingly difficult for us as a profession to define what is meant by normal birth. We seem to have problems in agreeing parameters of normality, especially around labour. This is probably because of the recent history of intervening unnecessarily in uncomplicated labour. It seems to me that what is seen as 'good birth' today is actually 'natural childbirth', not 'normal childbirth'. What do I mean by that? Well, natural childbirth, I would say, is allowing pregnancy and birth to proceed as nature decrees, and without intervention. This means that most will be successful, some will be damaged, and some will die — very much as childbirth is in the developing world. However, damage and death in childbirth is largely preventable in a developed society such as ours. That is why normal birth, which is the midwives' role, should take place within agreed parameters, and when those parameters have been breached, timely and appropriate intervention will rob nature of her morbid victory.

Choice

Another area that I think we should be concerned about is the choice agenda, and its implications for the midwife. 'Choice' is a political word of the day, and it will pass. In saying this I give my critics the opportunity to say that I do not want women to have choice, but want to nail them to the bed and do things to them. This is far from the case. I see choice as very important. What I am concerned about is the manner in which choice extends into the technical and professional aspects of what we do. Midwives, it seems to me, are often too ready to support choice, and forget that in supporting it they also have a duty of care.

This view is reinforced when I sit on the Conduct and Competence Committee at the Nursing and Midwifery Council (NMC). There I see good midwives who have not thought this through. They believe they should support women even if they choose the most inappropriate care, and they fail to safeguard themselves by consulting obstetricians and supervisors of midwives, and by failing to document decisions reached meticulously. If things go wrong and the woman then brings a complaint to the NMC, the midwife may find herself ultimately being deprived of practice.

There is much for the pregnant woman to have choice, but was choice ever meant to extend into those technical and professional areas for which we have been extensively trained, and for which we hold professional accountability? What a grey and fragile area this is!

I know that the secret of women being happy to take advice from midwives, appropriate to their individual circumstances, resides in the midwife-woman relationship. Of course there are midwives and women at the extreme, but generally midwives and women within their special relationship can come to a decision which serves the needs of choice, accountability, and duty of care. I could go on.

Working Conditions

I worked for some 35 years as a clinical midwife at Liverpool Women's Hospital, which sees some 8,000 deliveries a year. During that time I witnessed the joy of birth many thousands of times, sharing that moment with Liverpool families. I have also known the deep sorrow of seeing 14 women die in the attempt. I have worked with truly outstanding, remarkable midwives and doctors, and have been inspired by their skill. I have shared with them the unparalleled experience of normal birth, but also many catastrophic situations over the years. I have seen them almost walk on water in these most dangerous and dramatic situations, and have driven home after my shift at such times almost bursting with the relief and joy of success.

I was amongst the first married midwives to work in Liverpool, and then had my own children before the days of statutory maternity leave. Those relatively few of us who had children at that time were in uncharted waters. We had to leave work, and draw out our superannuation, drawing what we thought would be a line under our professional life, since at that time almost all midwives were single and worked full-time. However, after my children went to school I was allowed the new, and rare privilege of working part-time, which I did for many years as part of the first generation of educated women to juggle home, children and a profession.

Today's midwives may note with envy that I was able to have the choice of staying at home to rear my children, a choice open to relatively few women nowadays. This was because mortgages, when granted, took only the husband's salary into consideration, which meant that when the women gave up work all the essentials of living were affordable using the husband's salary. Today, though standards of living are higher, I feel anxious that because mortgages are granted taking both incomes into account, few women have the choice of staying at home for very long to rear their children. So much for liberation!

When I was at home with my children I missed midwifery tremendously, and it is true to say that I would have gone back without pay for the sheer joy of it. But I could not say that today because midwifery is practised in a very different, difficult, constantly changing, and pressurised NHS.

For a while I was content working part-time. Such an arrangement meant that I had the best of both worlds at home and at work. However, it was not without its problems. A common attitude towards those who worked part-time was that they were only there for the pin-money — they did not need any professional updating except the statutory refresher courses every five years, and indeed they were not as dedicated as their full-time counterparts, and certainly they had no aspiration or hope of promotion. For all my faults, that description did not fit me. I was professionally and politically aware and was keen to engage in all the innovations in practice which midwives became involved with, and to work any shift on any day, exactly the same as my full-time colleagues. Indeed, during this time I was a frequent lecturer on study days for midwives, and wrote chapters in textbooks.

I have always been an articulate woman who dislikes controversy but hates injustice even more, and over the years I found myself championing many local causes for midwives. I became involved in my branch of the Royal College of Midwives (RCM), variously as its chairman, secretary, treasurer, and most taxing of all as a steward. In this role I was able to support midwives through grievance and disciplinary procedures, and although I found this role very rewarding it was at times very distressing.

However Liverpool humour often sustained me. For instance, while helping a colleague one day I seemed to get my words mixed up, when at the delivery of his child a man said at the crucial moment: '*Oh, I do feel funny*'. '*Put your hands between your legs*', I said. Quick as a flash my Liverpool colleague said: '*It won't make you feel any better, but it will take your mind off it!*' Of course, what I thought I had said to the man was, '*Put your head between your legs*'.

On another occasion when I was hoping to have a cup of tea with colleagues the door bell rang, and a man said to me: '*Good morning, Sister. I've brought my wife for inducement. I was going to bring me ma with me. She's had twelve. Me father's a Roman Catholic and has no sense of rhythm*'. Can you imagine what a fun day I had with him and his wife, as I looked after her in labour?

However I must not paint a saintly picture of myself. Due to constant changes, pressure of work, inadequate staffing levels, or whatever, some days I felt I had horns and a tail as I tried to be a good shift leader on a labour ward which too often resembled a war zone. On such days I did not like myself, and I dread to think what others thought of me, as I suspect we all do when we have such days. However my experience has been that colleagues — themselves under pressure and understanding the stresses and strains which take place increasingly often — are very forgiving, and take the view that it is the pressure of work which is largely responsible for such behaviour. Not that this excuses it, but it does explain it. This is why those cups of tea together are absolutely vital: a time to put things right with each other and to discuss the things going on in our lives which may affect our work.

RCM Council

Aged 50, my family grown, and my parents dead, I felt I might have 10 years or so before retirement to do something for myself. I did not want to study for a degree. What use would that be to the profession at that age? If I were to work for a degree it would be for myself, and probably in medical ethics. My husband has always believed that I would have achieved more professionally had I not married and had children. Whilst this may be true, I actually wished to stay in the clinical area. What I did long for was some career progression for those who wished to continue as clinical midwives. Until recently there was none.

I had always had much to say, and held strong opinions, about most matters professional, and in common with most midwives I had always been good at airing those views in the tearoom. I though it might be more effective to do this where those views had some hope of being listened to, so I decided to seek election to the Council of the RCM. In order to do this I had to write a manifesto and do some serious reading. I was successfully elected, and it changed my life.

The papers for the first Council meeting dropped on my doormat in a huge bundle, which required very serious reading and consideration. My initial reaction was that I had made a big mistake, but I told my husband I must go to Council at least once, because I had been elected.

In London, I walked into the debating chamber of the RCM Council and saw all the faces and met all the people I had hitherto only seen in our journal *Midwives*. I heard the debate, the passion, and the diverse opinions, and I was hooked. I loved every second of it. I would advise midwives to have the aspiration of being actively involved in our professional body, the oldest and largest midwifery establishment in the world, which we should cherish.

The things that I moaned about in the tearoom which seemed to me to be easy to address in reality were not nearly so easy to resolve. I grew up politically and got so much more from my profession. I served my first term of three years, and almost on a whim put my hat into the ring for the Presidential election. I was successful, and began the most wonderful, fulfilling, exciting, and rewarding eight years as your President, representing you nationally and internationally at branch meetings, seminars, government departments, and palaces. What a privilege it was to represent a profession so well respected and so well understood worldwide! Everyone is touched by a midwife.

During this time I attended the 100th birthday of our Patron, the late Queen Elizabeth the Queen Mother, I had tea with her on two occasions, and sadly some years later I represented you at her funeral. I had lunch variously with the Queen and Princess Royal, and worked on the Council of The Kings

Fund, whose working President is the Prince of Wales.

Each year the Prince of Wales invites Council members of the Kings Fund and the great and good from London who work in the health service, to the King's Fund lecture at St James's Palace. On my first visit I sat in the throne room with red damask and gold leaf on the walls, the sun shining through open windows, listening to the soldiers marching and a band playing. What a contrast I thought, to my life yesterday morning when I was trying to run a hugely busy labour ward, and was longing for a cup of coffee. Sitting next to me was the President of the Royal College of Nursing, who said: *'You're not staying for lunch, are you? It will only be a couple of canapés and a glass of wine. I'll treat you to lunch at Fortnum, and Mason's'*. I thought: *'I believe I could get to like this lifestyle'*. Returning home to Liverpool later that day I travelled first-class (which was unusual because Virgin Railway was offering a special ticket for £14). What a remarkable day it had been! Sitting at my kitchen table, telling my husband all about it, and eating some shortbread, some crumbs fell on to my dress. Brushing them away with my hand, the dress felt very strange. I looked down and to my horror, discovered that I had been to all those places that day with my dress on inside-out.

During my time as president I travelled to Vienna, the Philippines and America. I also visited some 150 midwifery units to meet and talk with midwives in the workplace. It was an enormous privilege, and I like to believe that if a part-time clinical midwife from Toxteth in Liverpool could do this, then so can you.

In 2000 I was awarded a DBE (Dame Commander of the Most Excellent Order of the British Empire) for services to midwifery. I cannot begin to express the pride I feel in that award for myself and for midwives.

In 2004 my term of office as President and retirement from clinical practice came together; the Presidency because my term of office had expired, and my clinical work because I underwent major surgery and running around a labour ward on night duty and day-duty at the age of 62 years, was no longer an option.

However, three years later, I have done sufficient hours on issues related to midwifery to still be able to send in my intention to practise.

Epilogue

Do I miss midwifery? Yes, there is a huge sense of bereavement, and I find it difficult to think of my profession in which I have invested so many years marching on without me. However, I do not miss the exhaustion, frustration, constant reorganisation of the health service, staff shortages, and shift work; but the essential business of midwifery, and the wonderful, talented, generous spirited professional people who are the NHS of which you now form a part, I shall always miss.

Dear students, good luck. I wish you well.

Activity 11

1. Write an account of an inspirational mentor, teacher or role model who has inspired you and helped you get over your lows in midwifery.

References

DHSS (1970) *Standing Maternity and Midwifery advisory Committee (Chairman, J.Peel) Domiciliary midwifery and Maternity bed needs.* HMSO, London

DHSS (1986) *Report on Confidential Enquiries into Maternal Deaths in England and Wales 1979–1981.* HMSO, London

DH (1993) *Changing Childbirth.* DH, London

INDEX

A

Administration of Medicines 27
Admission 60, 73
Antenatal testing 67
Application 73
Autonomous midwifery practice 146

C

Caesarean section 86
Career opportunities 68
Careers 55, 170
Challenges 63
Changing context 138
Childbirth 57
Choice 192
Clinical environment 45
Clinical governance 123
Clinical setting 63
CNORIS 126
CNST 126
Coaching 45
Code of Professional Conduct 20
Communication 67
Competence 37
Complaints 129
Compromises 75
Conduct and Competence Committee 18
Confidence 37
Conflict 161, 170
Consensus development reports 101
Culture 161, 164

D

De-professionalism 171
Decision-making 66
Defensive practice 118
Demands 189

E

Economic bondage 155

E (continued)

Education 23, 59, 88
European Union Midwives Directive 63
Evidence 95, 100, 105
Evidence-based practice 95
Expectations 78
Experiences 71

F

Feedback 49
Femenist perspectives 151
Feminism 152, 158
Feminist backlash 157
Flying squad 185
Future perspectives 93

G

Gender roles 153
Government policies 144
Guidance 49
Guidelines 101

H

Health Committee 18
Hierarchy 172
Highs and lows 77
History 14, 55

I

Ideology 162
Implementation 107
Investigation Committee 18

L

Law 15
Leadership 168, 176
Learning needs 48
Litigation 117

M

Management 45, 166
Mentorship 39, 79
Midwifery Committee 18, 19
Midwives Rules and Standards 25
Multidisciplinary working 67

N

Natural childbirth 192
NHS 142
NMC 15
Normal childbirth 83, 192
Notification of Intention to Practise 26

O

Opportunities 161, 174
Options 72
Organisation 176

P

Partners 174
Partnership 66
Patriarchy 153
Personal developement 50
Physiology of normal birth. *See also* Normal childbirth
Policies 144
Policies and protocols 127
Policy 174
Political constructs 137
Pre-registration 23
Preceptorship 41
Preparation 74
Primary literature 100
Professional development 50
Professionalism 171
Professional networks 47
Professionals 166

Q

Qualitatve research 99

R

Randomised controlled trial 97

Records 27
Regulation 56
Responsibility 27
Risk 182
Risk management 123
Role models 47
Roles 175

S

Sacrifices 75
Search techniques 101
Self-reliance 38
Social constructs 137
Social enterprises 163
Social profile 140
Society 15
Staffing 169
Statistics 85
Statutes 13
Statutory Committees 18
Strategies 101
Supervision 28, 44
Support 48, 67
Systematic reviews 100

T

Technology 144
Tensions 173
Tools 39

W

Water birth 103
Welsh Risk Pool 126
Working 65
Working conditions 193